A^TR^HM^EE D

ROBBERY

ORGASM

ALSO BY JOHN MONEY

Hermaphroditism: An Inquiry into the Nature of a Human Paradox, 1952

The Psychologic Study of Man, 1957

A Standardized Road-Map Test of Direction Sense (with D. Alexander and H. T. Walker, Jr.), 1965

Sex Errors of the Body: Dilemmas, Education, and Counseling, 1968

Man and Woman, Boy and Girl: The Differentiation and Dimorphism of Gender Identity from Conception to Maturity (with A. A. Ehrhardt), 1972

Sexual Signatures (with Patricia Tucker), 1975

Love and Love Sickness: The Science of Sex, Gender Difference, and Pairbonding, 1980

The Destroying Angel: Sex, Fitness, and Food in the Legacy of Degeneracy Theory, Graham Crackers, Kellogg's Corn Flakes, and American Health History, 1985

Lovemaps: Clinical Concepts of Sexual/Erotic Health and Pathology, Paraphilia, and Gender Transposition in Childhood, Adolescence, and Maturity, 1986

Venuses Penuses: Sexology, Sexosophy, and Exigency Theory, 1986

Gay, Straight, and In-Between: The Sexology of Erotic Orientation, 1988

Vandalized Lovemaps: Paraphilic Outcome of Seven Cases in Pediatric Sexology (with M. Lamacz), 1989

Biographies of Gender and Hermaphroditism in Paired Comparisons: Clinical Supplement to the Handbook of Sexology, 1991

The Breathless Orgasm: A Lovemap Biography of Asphyxiophilia (with G. Wainwright and D. Hingsburger), 1991

The Adam Principle: Genes, Genitals, Hormones, and Gender: Selected Readings in Sexology, 1993

EDITED BY JOHN MONEY

Reading Disability: Progress and Research Needs in Dyslexia, 1962

Sex Research: New Developments, 1965

The Disabled Reader: Education of the Dyslexic Child, 1966

Transsexualism and Sex Reassignment (with R. Green), 1969

Contemporary Sexual Behavior: Critical Issues in the 1970's (with J. Zubin), 1973

Developmental Human Behavior Genetics (with W. K. Schaie, E. Anderson, and G. McClearn), 1975

Handbook of Sexology, vols. 1–5 (with H. Musaph), 1977

Traumatic Abuse and Neglect of Children at Home (with G. Williams), 1980

Handbook of Human Sexuality (with B. B. Wolman), 1980

Handbook of Sexology, vol. 6 (with H. Musaph and J. M. A. Sitsen), 1988

Handbook of Sexology, vol. 7 (with H. Musaph and M. Perry), 1990

Handbook of Sexology, vol. 8 (with J. Krivacska), 1994

THE ARMED ROBBERY ORGASM

A Lovemap
Autobiography
of Masochism

Ronald W. Keyes & John Money

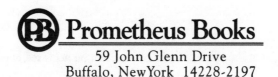

Prometheus Books

59 John Glenn Drive
Buffalo, New York 14228-2197

Published 1993 by Prometheus Books

97 96 95 94 93   5 4 3 2 1

Library of Congress Cataloging-in-Publication Data

Keyes, Ronald W.
    The armed robbery orgasm : a lovemap autobiography of masochism /
Ronald W. Keyes, John Money.
        p.   cm. — (New concepts in human sexuality series)
    Includes bibliographical references.
    ISBN 0-87975-856-2
    1. Keyes, Ronald W. 2. Masochism. 3. Psychosexual disorders.
I. Money, John, 1921–   . II. Title. III. Series.
RC553.M36K485   1993
616.85′835′0092—dc20
[B]   93-5868
                                                                                               CIP

Printed in the United States of America on acid-free paper.

To Pam, my childhood playmate

Contents

Foreword

There used to be a time, extending into the twentieth century, when families would hide one of their own members who was wasting away and dying from pulmonary tuberculosis (consumption). It was a disgrace to admit to having tuberculosis in a family member, for the wasting away or consumption of the body was considered to be a manifestation of degeneracy brought about by depriving the body of its most precious vital fluids. In the male, that meant semen depletion by excessive sexual activity, especially by masturbation. Germ theory, discovered in the 1870s, finally displaced the archaic semen-conservation theory as an explanation of the cause of tuberculosis, but it did not take away the disgrace of diseases attributed to sex. In the present era, AIDS is an example.

There are many instances in which attributing the cause of death to the AIDS virus (HIV) is evaded so as to spare the survivors the disgrace or shame of having to admit that their deceased member may have been homosexually exposed to the infection. Another present-day evasion is that of attributing death of a family member to suicide instead of to the syndrome of autoerotic asphyxiophilia. The shame of this syndrome is that the deceased, usually a teenaged or young adult male, dies in the course of a masturbation ritual. Incorporated in this ritual is a penalty for the sin of lust, namely the exhilarating danger of death-defying self-asphyxiation. In a split second error of timing, the noose fails to loosen, so that unconsciousness and death ensue.

Many, if not most, people are diffident about public disclosure of a defect, injury, or disease affecting the sex organs, and not altogether

9

without reason—disclosure may subject one to societal stigmatization. For instance, the very term *hermaphrodite* stigmatizes the baby born with ambiguous genitalia, and the parents as well. To have been born with imperfect genitalia is to bring shame and embarrassment, if not disgrace, to the family.

Public disclosure of a disorder or syndrome that affects not the sexual anatomy but sexual behavior may be conducive to not only stigmatization, but also to a societal response ranging from derision and disgust to condemnation, anger, and vengeance. Behavior that evokes such a response is popularly characterized as offensive, deviant, perverted, or criminal. The biomedical term is paraphilic. To avoid self-incrimination, people with a history of paraphilic behavior have sufficient reason to keep it quiet. Otherwise they risk the social penalties of disclosure, which range from being humiliated, shamed, and disgraced, to being censured, arrested, and tried as a criminal. Those whose sexual behavior, dreams, and thoughts put them at risk for societal reprisals use privacy, evasiveness, and self-censorship to restrict the amount of information that may safely be disclosed. Thus sexological science is deprived of access to information that will bring about fuller understanding of human sexuality and eroticism as well as the great diversity of its manifestations.

Personal information of a sexual and erotic nature might be disclosed provided total confidentiality can be securely and irrevocably guaranteed. No such guarantee is possible if the information is by law subject to mandatory reporting, as in the case of pedophilia, for example. Nor is it possible if an informant, having been arrested, is referred for sexological evaluation by either his own attorney or the state, under which circumstance the record of his evaluation may be subpoenaed by the court. Once a person has been sentenced for a sexological offense, however, or has served his sentence, the danger of self-incrimination from self-disclosure does not apply to information already publicly disclosed in the court record at the time of the trial.

This is precisely the history of the information autobiographically revealed in this book. The writer cannot be penalized a second time for what he writes about here, but it is nonetheless an act of very considerable social courage to have written it. There is no prophet to foretell whether the societal response will be vindictive and rejecting, or forgiving and ready to learn from the self-knowledge that the author has compiled for the benefit of sexology at large as well as for himself. His own benefit has been, in part, rehabilitative. Lacking any experience as a writer when first imprisoned, he took correspondence courses in freelance writing. At the same time he took up the study of sexology and, with much tutorial guidance by mail, perfected the vocabulary, grammar, syntax, style, and logic prerequisite to being the author of a sexological book. Despite the formidable obstacles of writing from the confines of a prison cell, the present volume is the outcome.

It is a remarkable volume in which the author's mirror, held up to family humiliations and punishments related to sexuality and masculinity in childhood, reflects them transformed into the erotic bondage and discipline of masochism in adulthood. It avoids jumping to the conclusion that the sequential relationship between the childhood and the adulthood experiences is causal. Instead, it formulates this relationship simply as chronologically sequential. This formulation allows for the inclusion of other contributing causes. In the present instance, another contributing cause is, almost certainly, being an affected member of a family pedigree positive for bipolar, manic-depressive disorder.

From the viewpoint of diagnosis, this is a book about paraphilia (from Greek *para-,* altered, + *-philia,* love). Though primarily paraphilic masochism (named after Leopold von Sacher-Masoch), the paraphilia is multiplex in its manifestations. The autobiographer as masochist is taunted and beaten into a state of erotic ecstasy by his dominatrix in the role of sadist (named after the Marquis de Sade). He is paraphilically turned on by images of himself as a sadist only in eroticized, noncoercive fantasies in which he paddles the buttocks of a capitulating, nubile female. He is sufficiently fixated on the form and appearance of the young adult nubile female that he characterizes himself as an ephebophile (from Greek *ephebos,* a postpubertal young person, + *-philia*) as well as a masochist. In addition he classifies himself also as a chrematistophile (from Greek *chremistes,* money dealer, + *-philia*), in recognition of his fixation on the basic paraphilic principle of incompatibility between erotic lust and affectionate love. This principle, as chrematistophilically expressed, dictated that his experience of erotic lust would be separated from affectionate love by always being paid for, whereas affectionate love would be separated from erotic lust, and not paid for. He was able to formulate the fit of all these paraphilic pieces into one multiplex paraphilic whole only after, while in prison, he became a student of paraphilia, using *Lovemaps* (Money, 1986) as his primary textbook. He maintained a voluminous tutorial correspondence with his mentor, who became the coauthor of this book.

His self-appointed laboratory exercise was introspective self-observation. In a daily log, he kept a private record of changes and sameness in the "mental videotapes" of paraphilic ideation and imagery that played in his dreams and fantasies, asleep and awake. He recorded their frequency and content relative to his mood swings and to the psychotropic medications sporadically prescribed for bipolar disorder. He recorded the occurrence of dreams and fantasies also in relation to erections, masturbation, and ejaculation.

The thematic content of his "mental videotapes" was predominantly spanking, with himself doing the spanking far less often than being spanked. His role was that of slave, totally subservient and obedient to his dominatrix, whose spanking of his buttocks would precipitate an otherwise unattainable state of superorgasmic, masochistic ecstasy. Prior to imprisonment, the virtuoso performances of his dominatrix were those in which his being spanked was contingent on his first committing an armed robbery and bringing the money to her in the getaway car where she was waiting for them to make their escape. Her ultimate act of domination was to report him to the police as a criminal wanted for armed robbery, admitting at the same time her own collaboration.

At the time the armed robberies were happening, he had blindly obeyed his dominatrix, and not questioned her as to the significance of armed robberies in her life. Thus he does not know whether her own personal lovemap was one of paraphilic sadism that reciprocally matched his own lovemap of paraphilic masochism. Nor does he know, alternatively, whether she may have spontaneously grown into the state, not uncommon among lovers, of collaborative adaptation between partners—a state akin to what is known by its French name as *folie à deux* (two-person folly). Either way, once the collaboration terminated with imprisonment, he experienced no mental replays of armed robberies. His paraphilic enslavement was to spankings, not robberies.

After several years in prison, in the context of chrematistophilia, as aforesaid, he was able to distinguish what he called fantasies of masochistic lust bondedness from those of nonmasochistic affectionate love bondedness. The possibility of a real-life test of the latter is thwarted, however, by the all-male prison environment. He is totally devoid of lust for any male, and is erotically indifferent to the male form. The real-life test of love bondedness, together with the real-life test of total rehabilitation, must await his release from prison.

No one, including the author/prisoner himself, can prophesy what the outcome of the real-life test of total rehabilitation will be. Incarceration itself, exorbitantly expensive for the taxpayer, will not and cannot have "cured" his paraphilic masochism. Autobiographical self-discovery in writing, irrespective of its benefits, will not guarantee that its author will be rid of the possibility of paraphilic relapse or partial relapse. Nonetheless it will serve to open a bridge of communication between its author and those professional sexologists who can be trusted to talk with him in a genuinely nonblameworthy, nonjudgmental idiom. That means that his personal sexologist will not be an adversary, insidiously accusing him of lack of motivation or willpower to suppress manifestations of his multiplex paraphilia.

Instead, the sexologist and he will form an alliance against the paraphilia. On the basis of today's state of the art, their strategy will resemble that used in epileptology, namely to keep the symptoms under control or in remission while maintaining vigilance against a relapse. Their joint strategy will include selective use of pharmacologic substances in dosages and for periods of time specific to individual efficacy.

The antiandrogenic hormones, medoxyprogesterone acetate (MPA; Depo-Provera®) and cyproterone acetate (CPA; Androcur®) are the pharmacologic substances with the longest history, beginning in 1966, of having been used in the treatment of paraphilias (Money, 1987). According to more recent clinical anecdotal reports, antidepressant, antianxiolytic, antiobsessional, and antiepileptic medications also may be sporadically beneficial.

Sexology owes a debt of gratitude to the author of this autobiography. Without the honesty of self-revelation like his, the true nature of enslavement to paraphilia will not become known, and the mythology of preference, choice, and lack of remorse will not be dispelled. Without a true understanding of the nature and phenomenology of the paraphilias, ascertainment of the where, when, and how of paraphilias, and of how persistently they become patterned in the brain and the mind, will not be possible.

The persistence of paraphilic patterning in the brain does not signify that it must be inborn. Like native language, it can be developed postnatally and, nonetheless, be persistent. That is the lesson of this book. It is to the rapidly developing brain science (brain chemistry) of learning and remembering that the book's writer and its readers may look for the next step in understanding what has here been so courageously revealed. That will yield, in a second step, eventually to an understanding of the development of sexological health and its impairment throughout childhood. Then will follow the third step of knowing how to promote sexological health and prevent its paraphilic impairment from the beginning. Prevention is the ultimate goal toward which this book aspires.

John Money
Baltimore
October 1991

References

Money, J. *Lovemaps: Clinical Concepts of Sexual/Erotic Health and Pathology, Paraphilia, and Gender Transposition in Childhood, Adolescence, and Maturity.* New York: Irvington, 1986; Buffalo, N.Y.: Prometheus Books, 1988, paperback.

Money, J. "Treatment guidelines: antiandrogen and counseling of paraphilic sex offenders." *Journal of Sex and Marital Therapy* 13 (1987): 219–23.

Acknowledgments

I thank John Money for his patience and faithfulness; the PEN American Center, for its monetary assistance; the Writer's Digest School, for teaching me the basic principles of professional writing; my father's help, irrespective of his stoical ideology; and Charles Milland, who provided the typewriter with which to type this book.

Introduction

Paraphilia and the Insanity Defense

Gregory K. Lehne, Ph.D.

Ronald Keyes's *The Armed Robbery Orgasm: A Lovemap Autobiography of Masochism* describes in detail his state of mind associated with the nearly two dozen armed robberies which he and his girlfriend committed in July and August, 1984. His trial attracted local and national attention, because he employed an insanity defense disclosing lurid details of sexual obsession and masochism. The Baltimore *Evening Sun* of April 23, 1985, ran stories with headlines like, "Jury to decide if sex obsession pushed man over edge," and quotes from Mr. Keyes's diaries and testimony about his sexual needs and activities.

I evaluated Mr. Keyes and argued in court that he should not be considered criminally responsible for his crime spree. I testified that he suffered from serious mental illnesses that impaired his ability to control his behavior. This defense was rejected by the jury. Although Mr. Keyes had no prior criminal history, he was sentenced to several concurrent ten-year terms of incarceration.

Mr. Keyes wrote this book during his incarceration and remains in prison as it approaches publication. It should be viewed not as an apologia, but rather as a primary source document produced by a psychiatric patient (in conjunction with an eminent sexologist) striving to make sense of his own life history.

I initially evaluated Mr. Keyes in November 1984. It was my clinical impression, then and now, that he suffers from two serious psychiatric disorders—a bipolar disorder, and the paraphilia of sexual masochism. The bipolar disorder involves endogenous mood changes including manic and depressive episodes.

The personal information that Mr. Keyes describes in this book is not essentially different from that which he discussed with me at the time of my evaluation, and which he presented in briefer form to the jury at the trial. The major change is that Mr. Keyes has become a self-educated expert on sexology and his own condition. He thus uses terms and a conceptual framework that he has learned from Dr. John Money, and which he did not articulate at the time of my evaluation. But his phenomenological descriptions of his experiences remain unaltered from his discussions with me eight years ago, and are remarkably similar to his symptoms reported in his prior psychiatric evaluations. There is also considerable evidence in existence prior to the robberies and his legal insanity defense that collaborate Mr. Keyes's account.

Mr. Keyes had been hospitalized for one month for treatment of symptoms of these disorders in 1966 at age twenty-two (an involuntary commitment following a suicide attempt). According to hospital records, the suicide attempt was precipitated by the breakup of a relationship. He was noted to be grandiose, with poor reality testing and judgment, and possibly an underlying schizophrenic condition. Sexual problems were also noted.

Mr. Keyes received outpatient treatment in 1972, 1979, and 1980. The admission note from his 1972 treatment described the presenting problem as "compulsive sexual behavior that is becoming increasingly necessary to patient and yet very disturbing because it causes him to lose time from work and makes him depressed. . . . Patient is obsessed with one sexual fantasy—spanking nude bottoms. When patient becomes depressed he is *forced* to do these things and feels guilty and depressed afterward. All energy is going into this" [emphasis in the original].

Unfortunately, the mood disorder from which Mr. Keyes suffered was not adequately or consistently treated with medication, although he had benefited from a period of treatment with lithium. Even more unfortunately, his sexological disorder was regarded as a manifestation of personality problems rather than being recognized as a specifically sexological obsession and compulsion—a paraphilia. Thus his story is a tragic one, because psychiatric and pharmacological treatment has been available for both of his disorders, and he had repeatedly sought out such help but never consistently received it. Perhaps the failure of professionals to treat him adequately is part of the reason that Mr.

Keyes has become such a student of his own sexological disorder.

Even today there is insufficient understanding of sexological disorders such as the paraphilia from which Mr. Keyes suffers. His book may be part of the process of educating the public and professionals, as well as those involved in the criminal justice system, to an improved degree of understanding. His rehabilitation has been entirely determined by his own self-study. However, his book also provides examples of incarcerated men with undiagnosed and untreated paraphilias who may be likely to reoffend following their release unless something is done to rehabilitate them.

Some paraphilias may be associated with illegal behavior, and thus they become mental disorders of particular concern to the criminal justice system. In certain situations I believe that a sexually obsessive and compulsive paraphilic disorder may be so overwhelming that the affected individual may not distinguish between right and wrong or be able to conform his or her behavior to the standards of society. This position is not yet generally accepted among mental health, forensic, or criminal justice professionals. Nor are insanity defenses often accepted by judges and juries if they are based upon a diagnosed paraphilic disorder.

The issue here is what we can learn from Mr. Keyes's case history that will allow the public to administer justice, protect itself, and also show appropriate compassion for individuals who suffer from serious psychiatric disorders.

The insanity plea embodies social compassion for unfortunate and afflicted individuals. It also allows for variation in the management of an afflicted individual that is not strictly in accordance with the nature of the crime. Thus, psychiatric rehabilitation or management may be one goal that is facilitated by acceptance of an insanity plea, but in other cases a longer period of detention than is strictly indicated by the criminal offense may be enforced.

In the past, the insanity plea was most likely to be used in situations involving extremes of mental retardation, brain damage, or psychotic conditions. But new knowledge of psychiatric disorders such as the paraphilias raises questions about broadening the understanding of diminished criminal responsibility or insanity beyond that which the law readily acknowledges.

Insanity and diminished criminal responsibility (i.e., guilty but mentally ill) are legal concepts that are defined differently in the various states and federal jurisdictions. The underlying concept is that criminal responsibility is diminished when the individual has significantly impaired judgment (the cognitive test) and/or inability to control behavior due to the presence of a psychiatric disorder at the time when the offense was committed. For example, a woman who is so brain damaged or retarded that she does not understand that her behavior is illegal or wrong may meet the cognitive test for diminished criminal responsibility. A man who is actively psychotic and hearing voices commanding him to perform an illegal act may not have the ability to control his behavior, and thus may meet both the behavioral control and the cognitive criteria for diminished criminal responsibility due to a psychiatric disorder.

Paraphilias rarely involve impairment in thinking so extreme that it can be argued that the individual did not know that his behavior was illegal or wrongful. Nonetheless, individuals suffering from a paraphilia often show significant distortions in their thinking. These include justifications of their own behavior as not being wrongful or not harming others. However, such individuals generally still recognize that others believe that their behavior is illegal, wrong, or harmful, although they may personally disagree with these social beliefs. Furthermore, they often attempt to conceal their paraphilic behavior from others, which attests to their knowledge of its illegality or wrongfulness.

In the case of Mr. Keyes, he was always aware that armed robbery was illegal and wrong. He did not justify his behavior to himself or others. In fact, the wrongfulness of the robberies was part of the reason that it became incorporated into the sexual scenarios he acted out with his girlfriend. Her ordering him to do something dangerously illegal and wrong was part of the process of her sexual domination of him. Thus, the cognitive test of criminal responsibility was not argued in the trial of Mr. Keyes.

The ability of an individual with a paraphilia to control his or her associated paraphilic behavior is the critical test of criminal responsibility. Paraphilias typically preoccupy thinking to the extent that the individual may be driven to achieve relief through sexual enactment. Such enactment can be in fantasy alone, perhaps with masturbation, or otherwise acted out in behavior. The acting out of a paraphilia can occur in a dissociative or trance-like state. Long-lasting periods of acting out, including multiple orgasms, are not uncommon. Once the acting out has begun, it is very difficult, if not impossible, to interrupt it without outside intervention. In extreme cases, the individual loses the ability to control his paraphilia-driven behavior. Thus the acting out of the paraphilia may not be stopped or deterred even in situations where detection or arrest is not only likely but certain.

Yet despite the lack of control over acting out, paraphilic rituals are very specific and are elaborated in an intricate behavioral scenario. If there is a specified target or situation for the sexual compulsion, then the lack of control is manifested only in situations involving that type of target or situation. Thus in some situations there may be excellent self-control in general or prior to the enactment, while in other situations the paraphilic urges overpower the affected individual.

Paraphilia, like bipolar mood disorder, is an episodic type of mental illnes. When a paraphilia is active, it strongly influences thought and behavior. When it is in remission, the afflicted individual may appear fully competent and responsible. Thus, a major difficulty in utilizing a paraphila in an insanity defense is that there may be no clear evidence of the mental disorder at the time of the psychiatric evaluation or the trial other than the patient's self-report. In such cases, the presence of the disorder may be inferred from the individual's self-report of his mental state at the time of the offense. In some cases it may be inferred from the pattern of offenses or corroborated with data from an impartial observer. Mr. Keyes's book provides ample evidence for readers to decide whether they think he was able to control his paraphilic urges, or whether they overpowered and controlled him.

There were several unusual issues involved in the insanity defense offered in Mr. Keyes's case. He suffered from two serious psychiatric disorders, both of which were relevant in evaluating his criminal responsibility for the armed robbery spree. Both of these disorders could be retrospectively documented for nearly twenty years before the robberies. These disorders could also be documented in his journal contemporaneously with the crimes. Thus, there was no question that he had preexisting psychiatric disability. He was not attempting to malinger or fake the psychiatric symptoms for his legal defense.

Both of these preexisting disorders significantly influenced his participation in the illegal behavior. In my opinion, Mr. Keyes was experiencing a manic episode associated with the bipolar disorder at the time of the robberies. It is common for people's behavior to go out of control during manic episodes. A sudden onset and high frequency of atypical behavior is often an indicator of a manic episode, although such behavior is not typically illegal. Thus, the influence of the manic episode can explain the sudden onset and high frequency of Mr. Keyes's illegal behavior, but does not explain why his mania was acted out through illegal behavior such as robbery instead of other behaviors (such as a credit card buying spree instead of a robbing spree). Mania reduces and may eliminate behavioral control, but is independent of the *content* of the behavioral acts. Mr. Keyes's past history was devoid of criminal behavior and provides no evidence of any prior predispositions to commit armed robberies.

The presence of mania was a less significant feature in Mr. Keyes's insanity defense than the presence of paraphilia. For an insanity defense, the law requires convincing evidence of a direct relationship between the mental disorder and responsibility for the illegal behavior. In Mr. Keyes's case, the paraphilia of masochism led him to be controlled and dominated by his dominatrix girlfriend. It was she who ordered him to commit the robberies as a prerequisite of masochistic sexual involvement under her domination.

The relationship with the girlfriend actually represented a *folie à deux,* a collusion based upon shared psychopathology. The "armed robbery orgasm" of the book's title actually refers to the paraphilic turn-on of the girlfriend as well as Mr. Keyes's own masochistic orgasmic sequel. Mr. Keyes's paraphilia led him to become fixatedly and compulsively involved in a masochistic relationship with the dominatrix girlfriend, not with armed robbery. The girlfriend's turn-on apparently was armed robbery or perhaps more generally ordering a man to engage in certain types of illicit acts for which she ultimately would punish him. Thus, in this case the jury could perhaps understand the difficulty Mr. Keyes had in controlling his sexual obsession. What the jury found difficult to understand in the insanity defense was the connection between sexual masochism and the armed robberies instigated by the dominatrix.

The girlfriend turned Mr. Keyes in to the police and testified against him. Thus she was able to act out her own pathology with the help of the criminal justice system—to get her man punished. Mr. Keyes is not full of anger or bitterness over his long incarcertion for a brief and atypical (for him) spree of armed robberies. In this book he is not attempting to present himself as wrongly punished. After all, he is the sexual masochist. In the final analysis, the criminal justice system became a partner in collusion with this couple to enable them to act out the grand finale of their reciprocal paraphilias.

A theatrical characteristic of all paraphilias is their tendency toward triumphant display and resultant self-incrimination. When arrested, men with paraphilias often confess to many, if not all, of their acts of illegal paraphilic behavior. This book is not a simple clinical description of Mr. Keyes's paraphilic experiences: it represents an unusually full display and disclosure, with substantial erotic overtones. In the process of producing this book, not only is Mr. Keyes educating all his readers, but he has also turned his tragedy of lovemap vandalization into an eroticized triumph, namely the public confession of his paraphilic syndrome.

Mr. Keyes has accomplished a considerable amount of rehabilitation during his incarceration by learning about his condition and writing this book. With or without imprisonment, in my opinion he never was likely to commit another armed robbery. The robberies were situationally determined by the influence of the dominatrix girlfriend. If she had not ordered him, I believe he would not have ever committed an armed robbery. Nonetheless his underlying psychiatric and sexological disability will continue to need careful monitoring and treatment to remain under control. He knows now, as he previously did not, where to turn for help, and what sort of help to obtain if threatened with a relapse.

Prologue

Outset of Discovery

It was the foreboding night of my arrest. For the first time in my awareness or experience, my erotic thoughts and genital arousal were aborted. Throughout most of my forty years, it seemed, I had been possessed by erotic imagery and orgasms.

Caged in the Baltimore City Jail awaiting trial, I began the only criminal incarceration of my life. While watching a video movie at the jail, I questioned why I had arrived there. What made me commit multiple armed robberies with my young dominatrix as a prelude to our sexual activities?

The movie we were watching starred James Garner. In it a man coerced his girlfriend into illegal actions with threats of punishment for failure. She failed to follow his instructions. Her cruel boyfriend scolded her, then removed his belt to strap her buttocks. Tugging her tight shorts down her shapely legs at his command, she lay down on the bed with her bare rump exposed. The whipping commenced and the video showed her grimacing face as he beat her squirming body with his leather belt.

A surge of erotic excitement suddenly permeated my body. Ambivalently, I experienced genital stimuation by that scene of a girl being lashed with a strap. That started my discovery of my perplexing sexuality.

The jail's psychologist eventually referred me to The Johns Hopkins Hospital. After several calls to secure an appointment at the hospital's

Sexual Disorders Clinic, I asked my lawyer to arrange for my transportation from the City Jail. Someone there possessed some knowledge about what had happened to me, and I depended on this appointment for the answers.

Actually, without my mistress's sexualized influences, I would have starved to death before committing armed robbery. Yet, I followed my lustmate into twenty-four eroticized armed robberies. Now, I'd need to explain to the specialist at Johns Hopkins what happened to me under her luring influence.

On November 15, 1984, I was transported to the Johns Hopkins Sexual Disorders Clinic. Dr. Gregory Lehne greeted me and my escort. Initially, I spoke only with Dr. Lehne. He probed into my past with pertinent questions, and I replied candidly.

Contrary to my prosecutors, who miscast me, I didn't care about a pending prison sentence. However, I yearned to know why I behaved as I did, and why I needed spankings by my dominatrix. What arcane force made me, at forty years of age, jeopardize my future by following my young dominatrix into criminal activity that I would never have performed otherwise?

After listening to fragments of my sexually unprecedented history, and my criminal behavior with my young mistress Dr. Lehne excused himself to phone John Money, Ph.D., professor of medical psychology, professor of pediatrics, and director of the hospital's Psychohormonal Research Unit. Dr. Money expressed interest in my case and asked to interview me.

Along with my escort but without handcuffs, I accompanied Dr. Lehne to the Meyer Building, Room 3–171 to visit Dr. Money. I pondered notions of escape, but I had no interest. My enemy resided within me— I couldn't escape it so easily.

My escort sat outside Dr. Money's office, and Dr. Lehne and I greeted the sexology expert. I shook hands with a truly interesting man in his most curious office. I was seated in a comfortable armchair, and graciously offered a cup of coffee, which I welcomed. Dr. Lehne seated himself to my left, while Dr. Money sat directly in front of me at his desk. He turned on a tape recorder, and Dr. Lehne commenced the interview by explaining briefly what had brought me there.

I sensed that Dr. Money possessed the answers to my sexually perplexing life, which consisted of inopportune penile erections, intrusively unacceptable erotic imagery and finally criminalized activity with my lustmate, followed by incarceration.

Tangentially, we traversed my sexually unconventional life. During my discourse with the doctors, I wondered why I didn't meet with Dr. Money on my visit to the Henry Phipps Clinic at Johns Hopkins in 1972. Perhaps I wouldn't be here today—under arrest.

Unfortunately, I lacked a sufficient vocabulary to explain what took place in my mind and body for the prior forty years. However, I determined to seek and discover my sexual quandary. After all, I had nothing to lose. Not even my life seemed important. It had been systematically yet inadverently vandalized, and by the very people and society who condemned me.

The diagnosis by Dr. Money, in addition to bipolar disorder, was a paraphilia of masochism. I knew little about either one of those uninvited conditions. However, I proposed to discover everything about these conditions that had brought havoc into my life.

Dr. Lehne inquired, "Have you read *Love and Lovesickness,* by Dr. Money?" I replied, "No." Obviously, I'd wasted my years of study in psychology attempting to discover my sexological problems. Thus, after my return to the Baltimore City Jail, I called my dear friend Nancy Jones and asked her to mail me a copy of *Love and Lovesickness* by John Money, Ph.D., and she agreed.

Inexplicably, I hadn't experienced any erotic fantasy or genital orgasm since the night of my arrest weeks earlier. That absence of familiar horniness perplexed me greatly.

When Dr. Money's book arrived, I read it avidly and repeatedly. There wasn't enough heat in the jail that winter. Yet, I allowed nothing to stop me from studying Dr. Money's book. Besides discovering about my sexual self, I realized that most inmates had paraphilias. However, they didn't understand their criminal acts to be related to their sexuality.

Had I not read his book, I might not be writing this book. It revealed to me who I really am, a question everyone inquires of themselves. During my punitive incarceration, I traced my masochism's onset to the significant incident that precipitated its deleterious effect on my life, academically, socially, economically, and erotically.

Criminally, my alluring dominatrix and I perpetrated twenty-four armed robberies, all for the sole purpose of facilitating our orgasms. We didn't do the robberies so much as have them happen to us.

Now you will read what caused me (and could cause any infant) to become a paraphile. This is the actual story of why I couldn't resist following my blonde-haired mistress through a damnatory course of eroticized armed robbery, straight up to the gates of a prison's division of corruption.

During my pernicious and useless incarceration, I commenced an extensive study of my masturbatory fantasy and orgasms. After each of my approximately seven hundred orgasms per year, I recorded the accompanying erotic imagery along with the interconnections to my childhood. Faithfully, Dr. Money helped me to discover the significance of orgasmic fantasies, imagery, and ideation. Historically, my erotic fantasy research is one of a kind.

1

Goddess of Lust
Onset of Fixation

The air that January 1983 was bitter cold, but I was so aroused by Connie's luring figure that I didn't feel it. As I drove home to my apartment, I wondered why a man of forty years, and with more available women than he could fuck in a week, had just solicited a lady prostitute. Why must she be twenty years younger than I am? What is this irresistible urge to worship her pussy and be enslaved by her?

Then I mused over Denise. I had been to bed with Denise and her sister together. I had had a third sister refuse to get out of my car until I promised to fuck her. I had licked every inch of their skin. I had fucked every orifice of their bodies. I had tied their limbs to the bed, and driven them mad with orgasms. I had spanked their bare behinds until they climaxed. Yet, I was going to capitulate to Connie, who would manipulate my masochistic lust with more power over me than I had knowledge of myself. This was no weakness of mine. It was an irrepressible power over me.

Denise, sister of my former girlfriend, was working at the 2 O'Clock Club on Baltimore's Block. Denise was also my neighbor and occasional bedmate. I had no idea that night that she would introduce me to a girl who would alter the course of my life.

As I sat on a bar stool at the 2 O'Clock Club speaking with Denise, I gazed around the club and observed the stripteasers. I stopped to stare at a voluptuous blonde sitting across the stage. Her alluring form beckoned me to stop. A surge of blood rushed into my penis. I couldn't move. I was spellbound.

I turned to Denise with a look of curiosity. "Connie's her name," Denise said. I asked her to get me a date.

The thought of meeting Connie made me tremble. It wasn't an ordinary attraction, for I didn't long to kiss her lips or have sex with her. I longed to fall at her feet and worship her body, especially her genitalia. When I looked away from Connie, I found her tantalizing image in my mind. She'd entered my mental stage, but without my consent.

Denise returned after making an after-work arrangement. Connie would accompany Denise home and visit me shortly thereafter. I was so full of erotic tension that I felt out of control. I had to be near Connie, and gaze between her inviting thighs.

After arriving at my apartment, I tried to recall the last time this masochistic feeling had overcome me. I guessed it had been about two years ago. While waiting for Denise and Connie to arrive, I drank whiskey. I was so stimulated by this goddess that alcohol didn't affect me. I was sexually intoxicated.

I heard the girls at the door of my apartment. Opening it, I observed Connie. She stood about five-foot-one, and weighed about 105 pounds. Mostly, she displayed wide hips, a small waist, and shapely legs. Tacitly, Connie's eyes spoke to me saying, "Now, you're mine."

After Denise went home, I gave Connie a hundred dollars to express my gratitude for arriving on such short notice. Since Denise had told Connie that I didn't desire sexual intercourse, my goddess of lust wanted to know what I expected of her. I asked Connie to play the role of a dominatrix.

Not all girls are right for this role, but I knew she was. Connie handcuffed my hands behind me and ordered me to kneel in front of my couch. My pants were off, and my engorged penis stuck out rigidly. Connie seemed delighted with her role of teasing me with her alluring body. She posed at the edge of my couch and directly in front of my face. Connie's cunt was sending my sexual brain into a turmoil of lust. Her shapely thighs were spread widely in front of my entranced eyes. She caressed her own skin tantalizingly. Soon my entire organism was aquiver, overwhelmed. As I stared at her captivating crotch, I saw her vaginal juices ooze from her labial cleft.

My erect penis was inflated more than usual. All of my senses were intensified. My visual perception was like that on an acid trip. I shuddered from the erotic energy permeating me. Domineeringly, my queen of lust warned me against moving. "I'll whip your ass so hard you won't be able to move," Connie said. Then, my brain recalled briefly that my mother and sister made the same menacing comments in my childhood, and Connie appeared much like my older sister.

Verbally, Connie teased me about viewing her vulva, and licking her labia. She ordered me to declare how much I wanted her body. She tormented me with desire for her, but refused to allow me satisfaction. Connie demanded obedience from me, and stated emphatically that she'd get it. With no rational way to explain it, this beautiful goddess of lust had put me under her spell.

Connie moved to the middle of the couch. She ordered me to drape myself across her luscious thighs. My oozing penis was lodged between them. Connie commenced spanking my bare buttocks fiercely. She smacked my skin with all the force she had. It burned like I was being branded with a hot iron, but I knew that the searing pain would soon be transformed.

In my masochized state, I experienced a metamorphosis. My organism felt a euphoria that transcended any drug in the world. Suddenly, I didn't want my darling dominatrix to cease spanking me. If I died at that moment, I'd die in erotic bliss.

Connie stopped spanking me when her arm reached exhaustion. She made it quite clear that she owned me from that night onward. Instead of resisting her imposed domination, I surrendered. She was fixed in my mind as my autonomy. Kneeling against the side of my couch as she dressed, I couldn't take my eyes off her. Before she pulled her panties up, Connie told me to look at her cunt and remember it.

With a commanding, but quite feminine voice, Connie told me that she'd call the next day. Then, she left me with a raging hard-on. Connie had forbidden me to masturbate with anyone in mind except her. In fact, I couldn't think of any woman except her.

Connie's wide hips, smooth thighs, full breasts, pretty face, and pear-shaped buttocks impinged upon my mind that entire night. By the time I climbed out of bed the next morning, I'd achieved about ten orgasms. I stumbled into my armchair in the living room and tried to make sense of the night with my blonde-haired dominatrix.

Then, my telephone answering machine received a call. My lustmate called to say, "Think about me, Ron, think about me."

Over the next three or four days, my mind was filled with Connie's slender waist. The mere memory-image of her voice swelled my penis. Incessantly, my mental stage posed me draped across her thighs being spanked. During the mental spankings by Connie, my penis would be rigid as a rod. I couldn't reason or resist her subtle sadism.

Occasionally I'd experience a nonerotic phase. Flashbacks occurred during these phases. Most of them were of childhood. The younger of my two sisters dominated me unmercifully, and frequently beat my buttocks and thighs with a stick or extension cord. Connie was her look alike.

That February it snowed. A wild party was in progress in an apartment upstairs. I was invited. Everyone was drinking beer. I noticed a familiar girl who lived close by. She had dark hair with a shapely but petite figure. She spoke with me and I discovered her name, Diane. Several hours later, I returned to my apartment. I drank whiskey and watched television.

Somewhere around midnight, I heard a gentle knocking at my door. My mind supposed Connie might be there, but it was Diane. She had a glass of vodka in her hand. I invited her in with great curiosity. She made herself comfortable. She had pure lust on her mind.

Diane told me that I made her horny. She'd been watching me leave and return to my apartment over the past six months. With feminine boldness she said, "Let's go to bed." Then, without hesitation, she raised her skirt.

I couldn't understand myself. I should have been able to ram my dick up her horny hole, but my penis didn't swell. I made the excuse that I'd had too much to drink. Diane accepted my lie of convenience. She went home with a promise to return.

When my door closed behind her, I sat in the dark. What caused a man's penis to swell? I wondered. Why couldn't I get a hard-on and fuck Diane? I screamed to myself. It was free and available, but I couldn't perform sexually. I cried in the dark. I couldn't tolerate my confusion, I wanted death. I recalled that my mother had handled problems that way: she'd wish the world would end, and that she would die. Consequently, I vowed to discover the reason for my sexual quandary, even if it killed me.

The next morning, I cleared the snow off my car. The phone rang as I came back into the apartment. I listened to the voice through my answering machine. It was Connie. I trembled in anticipation as I picked up the receiver and spoke with her. My penis inflated like a balloon. Connie inquired about the messages she'd put on my answering machine. My dominatrix also asked whether I'd seen other girls naked. Hesitantly, I spoke of my encounter with Diane. Connie was irate.

Shortly thereafter, I drove to pick up my mistress at her house. While driving back to my apartment, she ordered me to stay away from all other women. My erect penis was oozing fluid onto the inside of my jeans. I felt euphoric. My queen of lust made herself my sole orgasm facilitator. She instructed me to remove my jeans the moment we walked into my apartment. She also wanted the paddle and handcuffs. I performed as she commanded me.

Connie perched her naked body on my fur-covered couch. I knelt in front of my mistress. I gazed at her cone-shaped bust. Connie spread her shapely thighs widely. Staring at her luscious body sent my mind into an erotic frenzy. While kneeling in front of her, I was instructed to repeat that I would never look at any other girls, especially naked. Connie promised to spank me harshly if I disobeyed.

My vandalized brain acknowledged her warning. Then Connie made me stay in a kneeling position while she smacked my rigid penis. She ordered me to leave it alone. The congestion in my abdomen from the overflow of blood in my erection was intense. Connie's intention was to torment me sexually. Even though I weighed fifty more pounds than my mistress, I couldn't resist.

"Now I'm going to beat your ass. And you will obey me," Connie said vehemently.

I arose and draped myself across her thighs. My buttocks were at the mercy of my domineering goddess. She pounded my bare skin with a wooden paddle. Connie paused to warn me against disobedience. Then she smacked my rump roughly. Inexplicably, the torturous pain transformed itself. My head was light. My body felt euphoric. Tacitly I begged her to continue my spanking. That feeling of masochistic elation was superior to a ton of cocaine.

Connie ordered me to stand. She stroked my penis and squeezed my scrotal nuts. "I want your dick to ache until tomorrow," she said viciously.

While I was driving her home, Connie made me stop so she could buy some pot. She demanded a hundred dollars for her grass habit. Then I drove her home. Upon returning to my apartment, I drank whiskey to soothe the aching in my groin. My penis remained rigid all night.

I awoke in a state of genital stimulation. The stimulus of my burning buttocks sustained my genital arousal. I panicked. Although it's an incredible high, it renders my reasoning powers void. When I stood in front of my mirror, the welts on my backside induced more swelling in my aching penis.

The redness of my spanked buttocks triggered a memory-image flashback. I was driving along the coast of New Jersey. When I gazed to my left, I saw a teenaged girl with sunburn on her upper thighs. The redness in the proximity of her young buttocks entranced my sexual brain. I could hardly continue driving. My penis swelled instantly. When I reached Baltimore, I sought a prostitute to help me cope with my masochistic arousal.

My answering machine turned on. I heard Connie's voice. Swiftly, I answered. She wanted to know if I'd played with my penis. I assured her that it was as hard as it had been when I left her. Connie then permitted me to jerk off, but only with her in mind. She also stated that I'd be spanked or strapped once a week from that point onward. Connie wanted to assure her dominance. She owned me with a power that didn't allow me to resist.

That night, I went to the 2 O'Clock Club to see her. I sat with Connie for several hours. She was spellbinding. I spent a few hundred dollars. Somehow, there seemed to be a connection between my sexual arousal and spending money. I didn't know what it was, then.

Since I was a self-employed salesman, I made my own schedule. I traveled over a ten-state area. Connie's salacious image never faded from my mind. When I checked into motels, I called her. Connie warned me against hiring other prostitutes. She didn't allow me to visit go-go clubs. Connie was the only female I'd be allowed to look at, dressed or undressed.

I was possessed by this princess of lust. There was no modifying love. My autonomy was absent. Many nights I'd achieve ten orgasms, but only when Connie permitted me to have orgasms. On my mental screen would appear Connie's luring vulva. It caused me to ooze seminal fluid. I'd focus on the image of her pink pussy for several hours with her in many poses. Once I'd climaxed, I'd rest for a while. Then it would start over again.

When I'd call my answering machine, I'd hear her voice in a most provocative way. "Think about me, Ron," she would instruct. As her words impinged upon my ears, my penis would swell. The feeling was enthralling, but I wasn't in control of my life. I couldn't even imagine resisting her domination of my mind and body. I knew that she'd eventually destroy me, and I was helpless.

Strangely, I had no appetite for food. I felt no pain. I wasn't tired either. My salesmanship increased. My sense organs experienced the world with acuteness. Engorgement of my penis prevailed throughout the day.

Whenever I returned to Baltimore, I couldn't wait to see Connie again. It was not the longing and eagerness of lust, nor was it affectional love. My yearning to see Connie was beyond love and lust. It was an irrational need to reenact a childhood spanking. My vandalized childhood had become incorporated into my sexuality.

Connie was working at the 2 O'Clock Club again. After parking my car, I gazed into the book stores and strip clubs on Baltimore's Block. I carried enough money in my pocket to hire a dozen hookers for sexual intercourse, but my mental mistress wouldn't let me. Then I entered the 2 O'Clock Club. I observed Connie, and immediately my penis commenced oozing semen.

Connie interrogated me. Did I see any girls naked? Did I stare at any girl's breasts? How much money did I earn? Did I masturbate? Did I dare fuck another woman? Connie wasn't satisfied with my replies. She reached into my crotch. With her fingers, Connie pinched my swollen penis. Grasping one of my testicles, Connie squeezed it. A stream of semen gushed down my pants.

"Tonight, I'm going to teach you to obey me," declared Connie, as she instructed me to stare at her partially bare bust. "In fact, I'm going to whip your dick so much that it'll hurt to piss." Inexplicably, nothing mattered to me except staring at her stimulating body.

At the club, I spent several hundred dollars while sitting with Connie. After the club closed, we drove to my apartment. Connie was beyond beautiful. Her voice was captivating. When we arrived, Connie ordered me to undress, get the handcuffs, and bring her the strap. Helplessly,

I responded to her demands.

When my goddess of lust disrobed, I was again amazed at her perfect figure. I knelt in front of Connie, while she sat on my couch. She teased me with her luscious endowments. Parting her cunt lips, she tantalized me. I shuddered as my masochistic lust for her pervaded me. Connie's shapely thighs beckoned my lips and tongue. Her full breasts elicited my mouth to suck on them. I was sensually ecstatic.

Then Connie stopped tantalizing me with her body. She folded the strap. She lashed my aroused genitals repeatedly. She held the neck of my erect penis, then lashed the head of it. She beat my penis and scrotum until they were sorely red. Sadistically, she glowed. My sensitized penis oozed fluid steadily.

Dominatrix Connie ordered me onto the couch. I knelt with my buttocks extended. Connie commenced strapping my bare buttocks. She lashed my rump with all the strength she possessed. The piercing pain felt as though I were cut with a knife. Then my masochistic metamorphosis occurred—I was so stimulated that I was euphoric.

When Connie reached satisfaction with her discipline of me, she called for someone to pick her up. In my metamorphic state, I'm disinclined to function effectively. Irrespective of how I achieved my masochistic euphoria, it seemed beyond this world. Nothing mattered now, except indulging the stimulative images of my brain. During masochized imaging, I achieved an orgasm each hour of that night. I couldn't label it masturbation, for I rarely used my hand.

Mostly, my mental images consisted of buttocks. I'd image them extended, exhibited, and redly spanked. Mental dialogue impinged upon my mind. "Please don't whip me, mama" caused ooze to escape from my erect penis. I'd image specified teenaged girls kneeling at the edge of their beds. I'd fantasize their vulvar cleft peeking from between their thighs. A fictive father or brother stood behind her and strapped her naked buttocks fiercely.

Occasionally, my masochized fantasies would reenact scenes from my terrorized childhood. My mother swung an extension cord sadistically across my thighs, buttocks, and genitals. "I hate you, you little brat, you're just like your father," she'd utter, and continue to whip me as though I represented her sacrifice. She vandalized my developing lovemap, and that impaired my lover-to-lover bonding forever.

Finally, when orgasmic exhaustion overwhelmed me, I rested. I awoke several hours later in masochistic tranquility.

For the next three months, Connie subjected me to weekly spankings. I capitulated as though life had no other meaning. Connie and I shared no genital interaction. In fact, I can't recall ever touching her with my hands. Yet I'd sell all that I possessed to lie across her thighs and be spanked again. Truly, I wished that I had a free will.

Then, without notice, Connie didn't contact me any more. She stopped working at the 2 O'Clock Club. I felt disoriented. I needed another masochized fix. Yet, I hated my dependency on her. Although Connie abandoned me physically, her provocative image remained in the furnishings of my sexual mind.

I felt an impinging urge for intense genital stimulation. I'd visit Baltimore's Block from afternoon until the clubs closed. The femininely visual stimulation incited masturbatory fantasy. The stripteasers would exhibit an arm, ankle, hip, thigh, nose, buttocks, or hair that would match an image in my sexual brain. Then, I'd spend the night in eroticized fantasy. Almost any long-haired blonde evoked mental imagery of Connie.

I'd perform all activities with an erection or pending erection. My masochistic preoccupation might be welcome if I didn't live in an economic, legally oriented society with deleterious religious and antisexual proclivities.

I concluded that only those who don't have my type of sexual condition claim possible resistance to it. When my paraphilia of masochism vied for expression, it bypassed my consent. Since it resides in my brain, and my brain controls my organism, I was helpless to resist. Fortunately, my sexual condition was not a predatory one, like raptophilia or erotophonophilia.

One month after losing contact with dominatrix Connie, I sat watching TV. From the visual stimulation came the urge to indulge erotically. I craved experiencing intense stimulation of mind and body in orgasm. Again I drove to Baltimore's Block as though entranced.

While seated in a club staring at the stripteasers, I overheard an interesting conversation. One of the strippers told another stripper about a customer who asked to be spanked after their coital activity. They wondered why a man would want such a crazy thing. Suddenly, an uneasy feeling overcame me, as though they knew I was a man of that kind.

Then I walked into the Villa Nova Show Bar. Donna, a sexy blonde, was dancing on stage. Her image corresponded to erotic imagery in my mind. I watched her wide-eyed. Her hair, thighs, and wide-hipped body entranced me. When she walked off the stage, I ordered a drink for her. I solicited Donna's services for after work that night. I gave her funds for a taxi.

While driving home, I pondered the reason for prostitution being illegal. I supposed that a female has every entitlement to charge a male for genital interaction, After all, it's her body. It seemed that the law against prostitution was designed to protect men, and dominate women. The male fucks the female, and she's stuck with a possible pregnancy. That's inconsiderate of the possible offspring. Perhaps the male should pay a possible child-support fee. I paraphrased the law to read, "If you charge me to fuck you, I'll put you in jail." I wondered why women tolerate such an unjust law, especially when they can defeat it by closing their legs until it's changed.

Donna arrived about 2:45 A.M. She wore a pretty white dress. Donna perplexed me greatly. Irrespective of the hundreds of girls I've copulated with, I didn't desire copulation with her. I longed to stare at her vulva. Donna accommodated me. She raised her dress, and lowered her panties. Donna sat at the end of my couch, and I stared between her thighs. I gave her a hundred dollars. There seemed to be an entrancement between her cunt and my eyes. I handed her another hundred dollars to continue. We talked, but my gaze remained constant. Then I bought more viewing time with a third hundred dollars. Donna sat with her knees up and thighs open; I couldn't withdraw my stimulated gaze.

I wasn't obligated by the typical male ideals that forbid the idealized man to enjoy a woman in any way but in sexual intercourse. Furthermore, I'm glad that there are many women who revel in having a man merely enjoy their physique with his eyes.

Several hours later, I shared breakfast with Donna. When she went home, I felt wonderful, but perplexed. Her value to me had been more than the three hundred dollars she cost. The tendency to spend money instead of persuading Donna to show me her pussy freely is what perplexed me. Otherwise, I was quite satisfied.

Subsequently, I solicited dozens of hookers. Mostly we'd indulge coitally. I conferred with several of them about playing the role of a dominatrix, but they were hesitant. Unfortunately, most women are accustomed to being dominated instead of being dominant. Nonetheless, coital activity didn't produce optimal orgasm, which is what I needed.

One afternoon, Donna left a message on my answering machine. She'd thought about playing the dominatrix. Donna said, "I think that I can do what you want." Unfortunately, my sexual brain didn't image her in that role. Donna was only a partial match to my vandalized lovemap, which made me suppose that I had some choice in calling her to play the dominatrix.

Meanwhile, Diane discovered one of my erotic zones from Denise. Diane was determined to be my bedmate. She arrived at my front door with a request for a beer. I invited her in and filled her request. She had no qualms about telling me of her intentions. Diane arose from my couch grasping the hem of her skirt. "Look, see, I shaved my pussy for you," declared Diane, as she exhibited it to my lusty eyes.

Suddenly, a surge of blood engorged my penis. I carried Diane to my bedroom. Spreading her thighs, I visually indulged her shaven vulva. Then, I pressed my lips against her labia. Diane was eagerly reciprocal. She longed for me to stroke the inner walls of her vagina with my swollen penis. Oozing, it penetrated Diane with passion. I pinned her arms down by holding her wrist against the mattress. My thrustful penis and pelvic motion drove her mad with orgasm. Forcefully, I pumped her voracious vagina. My sexualized energy didn't wane.

After several hours of vaginal, oral, and anal copulation, I collapsed in orgasmic afterglow. Diane endowed me with the title of being the best she'd ever experienced. Yet, I was satisfied only partially. Diane possessed only one allurement that aroused me sexually. Thus she would never be anything more than an episodic lustmate.

Eventually, I stopped going to work. Nightly, I'd visit Gail's Go-Go Club, which was in my neighborhood. There was one girl who conveyed an irresistible charm, but her effect was nonerotic. Hourly, I'd watch Mary dance. When I returned home, though, I'd still have erotic fantasies of Connie. My sexual brain demanded optimal orgasm from being spanked. Connie was absent, but not without influence.

Finally, after two months of watching her dance, Mary greeted me. I was delighted with her. Mary was enjoyably smart and pretty. Mostly, I enjoyed the lack of stimulation, genitally. Mary's genitalia did not matter to me, but I didn't know why. What was the allurement which Mary held for me? Why couldn't my genitals swell for her instead of dominatrix Connie? My questions remained unanswered.

For the next couple of months, Mary took me out to dinner once a week. She proved to be the most pleasant lady I'd known. Mary respected my accumulated knowledge and empirical experience.

I dreaded the day when my masochistic lust would summon me to submit, and divest me of my pairbond with Mary. To facilitate my deteriorating life, I drank a quart of whiskey daily. I didn't know what to do, nor did I have anyone to turn to. My genitals wouldn't swell under the aegis of anything but masochistic images. I longed for death to deprive my masochism of another victory.

It was December of 1983. Daily, I'd imaged Connie since the moment I observed her eleven months earlier. Even in absentia, Connie facilitated all of my paraphilic orgasms. Although I reveled in my nonerotic partnership with Mary, in her proximity I could experience neither penile lust nor fantasy. I yearned to replace Connie's imagery with imagery of Mary, but changing my paraphilic imagery was impossible.

As a Christmas gift, Mary presented me with a blank journal book. Since I already recorded the daily events of my life in a journal, I used Mary's gift to write about my distorted partnership with Connie. I was perplexed about my masochistic lust and where it might lead me. Compulsively, I felt the urge to record the irrepressibly bizarre events of my masochistic life.

One evening a few nights before New Year's Eve, I was in my apartment seated in my recliner. My television was on, but all other lighting was off. I heard a key being used to open my front door. My dominatrix stepped into my apartment. She wore a pair of black boots with high heels, a black leather skirt, and a black leather vest. Her breasts jutted alluringly, and her blonde hair glowed in the dark. Moreover, her proportionately perfect thighs enthralled me. Then, uncannily, her voice enslaved me.

My penis swelled instantaneously, and commenced oozing its fluid. Connie demanded money for her narcotic habit. I was reluctant to fund her attachment to illicit drugs, particularly since I couldn't work or think correctly in my masochized state of mind. Connie had only her own interest on her mind.

"OK, if you won't do it the easy way, I'll make you do it the hard way," Connie said, cruelly and sadistically. "Now give me your belt and take your pants off."

If I could have said no to her I would have. If I had possessed the choice of resistance, I would have exercised it. I found my flesh to be resistant to my mind. Although Connie weighed only 105 pounds, standing only five feet and one inch tall, she ruled me as though she were a giant. Therefore, at forty years of age, verging on monetary ruin, I handed my belt to Connie.

"I'm going to teach you not to refuse what I want," she snarled menacingly, as she ordered me to bend over the front of my couch. "Keep your hands off your dick or I'll beat that too."

Raising the leather belt high, she lashed my bare buttocks with all of her strength. I submitted to her like a naughty child. I was without volition. The stinging from the belt pierced my flesh and permeated every cell of my organism. My own masochism made me endure her angered battering of my buttocks. And I couldn't stop it.

The more Connie welted my buttocks, the greater the quantity of penile fluid that oozed and drooled on the floor. Then it happened again! Somehow there is no pain, but only masochistic ecstasy. I can't utter the words to have her cease strapping me. Eventually, she thinks that I've had enough punishment and stops beating me. I'm in another realm, but she doesn't know that.

My dominatrix collected her money, procured under duress. She threatened me with more punishment if I didn't find a means to support her. After she had departed, her dominatrix's image stayed with me. During that period, masochized lust kept my penis erect and insensitive to any external pain. It stayed as hard as a board.

As I lay on my bed, the masochistic scenarios replayed on my mental screen. The searing pain in my buttocks was my orgasmic facilitator throughout that night. My first orgasm felt as though my internal fluids were gushing through my urethra, the stimulation almost intolerable. My head jerked and my limbs twitched with sudden movement. My eyes rolled in their sockets. Then, my entire organism shuddered, quaked, and quivered. Finally, I sensed an orgasmic afterglow pervade every inch of my mind and body.

Briefly I rested, but my penis remained engorged. Then, in my masochized imagery, Connie's vulva appeared. Penile fluid began oozing again. I ejaculated eight more times that night.

Connie had ordered me to earn money for her. I obeyed her. I visited the East Mall near where I lived. There a salesman was selling carpet shampoo to passing shoppers. I asked him about the price of renting space. He directed me to the Mall Exhibition Company. I discovered that I could rent a space for three hundred dollars at the next exhibition, scheduled for the following week. I decided to sell polishing cloths, which would polish anything.

My mistress was pleased with me. She demanded to visit my exhibition stand, and to collect money. I was willing to satisfy my dominatrix whatever the cost, though I didn't understand why.

During the first day of the exhibition selling was great. I worked from morning till night. I collected four hundred dollars in profit. At the end of the day, I visited Mary at the club where she danced. I needed a few beers, and I longed to speak with Mary. My earnings for the day at the mall made me feel proud of myself.

While watching Mary dance, I pondered many things about my behavior. I knew my earning potential. Why didn't I save any of my earnings? Some men gamble their money away. I spend it on women, compulsively. I can't discover why I do it, nor how I might be helped.

Mary sat with me during her twenty-minute break. She was interested in my success at the mall. No masochistic feelings emerged. I felt like a normal man with Mary. Thus, it seemed that Mary elicited my love, and Connie my lust, albeit a distorted lust.

The next morning, Mary arrived to sell my polishing cloths with me. I gave her a percentage of each sale. Mary's enticing body lured the customers, and sales were prolific. She dressed in a most provocative manner. Her sexy voice couldn't be resisted. I had found a wonderful partner. By the hour when she departed for work, she'd earned a profit of a hundred dollars. Mary went to work elated.

In the evening, Connie arrived while I was selling. She inquired about sales in the mall. After bragging about my sales, I gave her $200. Connie promised that since I had worked so hard for her, she would let me view her luscious pudenda. Nothing else mattered to me. I could kneel between her thighs viewing her vulva forever.

Mary and I worked well together that week. The flow of our money exceeded $3,000. Connie didn't like Mary's participation but the money made her ignore Mary. Besides, Connie knew that a spanking would make me do anything, and she was right.

Since there was another mall exhibition in York, Pennsylvania, during February, I planned to attend. I anticipated good sales, for there was scheduled an automotive show in the York Mall at the same time.

To assure herself that I'd work hard, Connie put me across her lap for several spankings before I left for York. The night before I departed, Connie arrived to assert her dominance over my mind and body. Obediently, I handed her a wooden paddle. Removing my pants, I knelt in front of my goddess of lust. She leaned back on my couch spreading her shapely thighs. Masochistically, I stared at her luscious labia without motion. My entire body was aroused, especially my genitals. My penile fluids oozed as she tantalized me with her captivating crotch. Rational thoughts were replaced by paraphilic trance.

Connie warned me not to look or think about another woman. She demanded to know my whereabouts at all times. She instructed me to sell and earn extra money for her. I was to call her each night after work. Then I'd be allowed to achieve orgasms, but only while imaging her. My dominatrix threatened me with harsh punishment for any disobedience to her.

My paraphilic lust permeated every cell of my being. Connie's paraphila and my paraphilia reciprocated each other, lovelessly. Warning me not to lick her, she pressed her vulva to my lips. "I'll let you lick it when you return," she said, teasingly.

By my own volition, I do not choose to be spanked, especially at forty-one years of age. It was without my volition that my penis swelled in proximity to Connie. Without my consent, my penile fluids oozed while kneeling in front of her. I didn't volunteer to resist licking her vuluptuous vulva. While serving in the army, I had discovered how to overpower men who were twice my size, but I could not overpower the effect of this goddess of lust. Why couldn't I rape her? Why couldn't I be the one to spank her into submission? I discovered that no amount of logical reflection would overcome or resist the ungoverned lust of my paraphilia.

Connie ordered my aroused and trembling body across her lap. Tucking my oozing penis between her thighs, she positioned my buttocks for a spanking. The wooden paddle stung as it pounded against my bare behind. Striving to impress her will upon me, she paddled every curve of my rump.

After pausing to rest her exhausted arm, Connie warned me to be still while she used her fingernails to inflict more domination. Across my enflamed buttocks, Connie dug her sharp fingernails into me.

Uncannily, I longed for more punishment. My mind and body were once again transported into another realm. My masochistic euphoria permeated every cell of my organism. Dying across her lap would have been my ideal death. Disconcertingly, I actually felt comfortable in the throes of her punishment. But I was not myself. I was another self.

When Connie speaks domineeringly, I capitulate. I arose from her lap and stood directly in front of her. Grasping my erection with one hand, she smacked the head of my penis with her other hand. Then, she scratched my helpless penis with her tormenting fingernails. Mentally, I screamed for more penile torture.

"Do you want this in my mouth?" asked Connie, cruelly. I couldn't answer. Then, she put the glans of my penis between her teeth. She dug her teeth into the flesh with sadistic delight. She chewed my penis roughly. I couldn't move. She swallowed some of the fluid from my penis and paused to examine the effect of her bite marks on it. My erection jutted forward as though it yearned for more.

While Connie dressed, I watched in a trance. She reminded me not to masturbate without her body on my mind. I was to obey and think only of her. Didn't she know I couldn't do anything but think of her? She was my goddess of lust.

Since my mind and body were in an intense frenzy of masochism, I went to bed that night with the lust of Connie pervading my mind. My mental pictures were so vivid that they replaced my actual world. I felt as though I was having an out-of-body experience. I existed only in my mind and its masochistic imagery. The only moments of actual sensation occurred with each orgasm. Otherwise I experienced only my mental theater.

Next morning, when I arose to drive to Pennsylvania, my body, sheet, and blanket were saturated with semen. I felt as if I had ingested several hits of speed. In my hallway mirror, I saw the bruises, scratches, and redness from the punishment Connie had inflicted on my bare buttocks. The mere reflection of my buttocks in the mirror swelled my penis. But Connie's domination, in absentia, made me dress and go to work.

My reflexes and awareness drove my car, but my mental pictures were of my dominatrix. My self was divided. My penis functioned according to my masochistic imagery, while my sense organs drove my car. At least that's how my being felt.

After reaching my motel room in York, Pennsylvania, I achieved several more orgasms. Later, I attended the mall exhibition. My selling was the same as my driving had been. I functioned in two realms. My mind imaged lustfully, while my brain sold my polishing cloths.

I sensed that the customers within the mall viewed me differently, just as I viewed them differently, especially the shapely young females. Many women looked at me as though they knew my body and genitals were in a state of lustfulness. Then, one woman leaned forward and said, "You look horny as hell, do you want to go to bed?" I was dumbfounded by her lusty assertiveness. She had no way of knowing that my eroticized state didn't have anything to do with genital interaction or coitus. My lust functioned under the aegis of masochism, not coital activity. Her vagina or mouth would be only the receptacle for my orgasm.

My pockets were full of money by the closing of the mall that night. Weirdly, I disowned the money which I had earned. As I drove back to the motel, I pondered my concept of money and earnings. In hindsight, it pertains to an incident during my early childhood. My misguided mother took my paperboy earnings from me when I displayed my delight in the money by tossing the dollar bills into the air. The distorted connection between the money and my lust occurred when she thrashed me with a stick, for my genitals swelled to protect me from the painfulness of her punishment. As I would eventually learn, my masochized lovemap took on a secondary paraphilia, otherwise known as chrematistophilia, the money-dealer paraphilia. My genital lust and its manifestation is interconnected with my dealing with money.

Connie had called the motel and left a message. I returned her call and told her about the money. My earnings did please her. She interrogated me about my behavior. My penis swelled from her voice inflection over the phone. Images of being draped across her lap while being spanked by her pervaded my mind. Warning me not to think of any girls other than her, she allowed me to masturbate. That entire night was spent in masturbatory fantasy.

During the next day, I couldn't concentrate on selling my product. My paraphilia had consumed both my mind and my brain. Then an idea, facilitated by my paraphilia, occurred to me. I hired two teenaged girls to sell my product at the mall exhibition. Their sales were prolific. I reported my hiring the girls to sell for me when I called Connie.

My mistress didn't mind the girls as long as they made money for her.

The two teenaged girls worked for me throughout that week in the mall. Connie's blonde hair, full breasts, and pink pudenda pervaded my mental screen incessantly. By the end of the week, the feeling in my buttocks from Connie's spanking me had faded. Frustrated, I longed to feel the sting from Connie's paddle again. Then, and without my consent, my ephebophilic lust took center stage. My longing was transferred to the two teenaged girls. I yearned to gaze between their shapely legs.

2

Goddess of Crime
Onset of Armed Robbery Orgasms

I was seated in my armchair watching television, anticipating Connie's possible phone call. I had not seen her for some time. Then, my answering machine received a call. I listened to the voice. It was my mistress. Reactively, my penis swelled, and my entire body intensified.

"Ron, have you been thinking about me? How would you like to look between my legs? You know, I expect you to obey my rules whether I am available or not," Connie said, domineeringly.

Barely could I tolerate the hour before Connie arrived. My masochized brain was in a turmoil of anticipation. Finally, after several months of mental anguish, Connie arrived to prod my masochism again. I wondered why I needed this distorted lust, which only Connie could satiate.

Entering my apartment, Connie appeared strikingly beautiful. She wore a black leather miniskirt. Her gold blouse caressed the shape of her bountiful breasts. Teasingly, she raised the hem of her skirt while seating herself on my couch. Spreading her shapely thighs, she demanded that I kneel in front of her luring legs. She tugged her black panties to her knees and tantalized me. The mere visibility of Connie's labia induced a flow from my inflated penis. I could have knelt entranced, by Connie's cunt, forever.

Inserting her fingers into her moist vagina, Connie continued to entrance me. She teased me with her luscious form, and reveled in the power she exercised over me. I couldn't move.

"If I tease you enough, will your dick squirt without playing with it?" inquired Connie, as she moved her panting pussy closer to my eager eyes. "Besides, I'm not letting you jerk off; you must come by staring at my pussy."

Tantalizing me with alluring motions, sexy gestures, and impinging words, my lustmate sent me through the throes of paraphilic lust. While I was experiencing an unequaled euphoria, Connie ordered me to ejaculate. Then, after slight pelvic motions, I felt my sperm gush from my subjugated penis. My orgasm shuddered every cell within my body. Drained of intrapersonal energy, I collapsed on my carpet.

Connie was sinisterly satisfied, for she even controlled the spurting of my sperm. While I was recovering from orgasmic exhaustion, Connie declared that she'd move in with me soon. I was pleased and frightened, for I didn't think my body and mind could endure her continued presence. Yet, I didn't want to be without her sexual stimulus ever again.

Before going home, Connie instructed me to pick her up in the morning to go to a flea market. I didn't know what she planned, and I didn't care. Being with Connie was all I cared about.

In the morning, we went to the flea market together. I was to sell polishing cloths there. My capacity to earn money as a traveling salesman had perished. My masochized mind and body vied with selling polishing cloths. It demanded expression, irrespective of my economic welfare.

Connie wore a brown miniskirt with a tightly fitting blouse. Her presence made it hard to concentrate. Thus, I couldn't promote my product with efficiency. Yet, in proximity to Connie, my brain had no difficulty swelling my penis.

Later, upon our arrival at my apartment, I yearned for an orgasm. Although I didn't want to endure the masochistic ritual of being spanked, there was no better way. Paraphilic sexuality isn't logical.

Maintaining her domination, Connie ordered my jeans off. She motioned for me to drape myself across her bare thighs, with my engorged penis hanging between her inner thighs. The pounding of her paddle stung intensely. I cringed, and suddenly my masochistic metamorphosis began, permeated my senses and transported me into another realm.

Sadistically subjugating me, Connie forewarned me of her living with me. Ambivalently, I longed for the masochistic stimulation, but sensed its foreboding implications.

Bemused, I questioned myself. What is this fortuity of life which coerces me to abide by this irrepressible existence of masochism? Was it transferred in the genes of my mother or father? Did I encounter some inexplicable contaminant at my birth? Why aren't my brothers and sisters equally plagued? Must I atone from some Biblical sin I know nothing about? Perhaps there was one incident that triggered an ominous sequence in my developing brain. My musing arrived at only one conclusion. Life is a sequence of accidents, and no one is at fault. Actually, we're all victims, one way or another.

A few weeks before Connie moved into my apartment, I was approached by three women sexually. Janet would have forked her thighs for me, and squeezed the sperm from my penis, but my penis didn't swell with her, although, ideally, Janet was beautiful. I could have copulated with Terry throughout any day that her husband worked. My neighborhood reputation had elicited her coital interest. Unfortunately, there was no image of reciprocity to swell my involuntary penis. Doris had a boyfriend, but she couldn't stay away from me. Her boyfriend wanted to kill me.

My sexual prowess instilled intense jealousy among the men who worked for the maintenance division of the apartments where I lived. But my dominatrix was the only one who could sway me in any way.

Ominously, in April 1984, Connie called me. Her intended move was to occur that day. Anxiously and apprehensively, I drove to collect her three cats, her baggage, and Connie herself.

I watched while Connie unpacked. She appeared placid and serene. I couln't say the same for myself. My masochized brain tormented me. Reverberating within my mental discourse was the insidious message that Connie must dominate me. Autonomy and nonautonomous feelings jostled for center stage in the mental theater of my deteriorating life.

A small park separated my apartment from a grocery store. I strolled to that grocery store with Connie. On our return trip, I held a bag of groceries with one hand. Connie held my other hand. There was a fraction of affectionate love in our partnership, and for the first time I felt it. An attenuated love is what I felt, and only briefly.

That evening Connie allowed me to enjoy her in copulation. That was an event for which my brain hadn't rehearsed. Connie was slowly responsive, as I caressed, kissed, mouthed, and tenderly nibbled literally every inch of her satiny skin. Connie's eyes remained closed as though erotic fantasy pervaded her brain. My genital excitement elevated in stages. Connie was the quintessence of my ideal of femininity.

Gazing at Connie's flared labia, I had a premonition of the beginning of my doom. My erect penis felt numb with hardness, as it entered my goddess of lust for the first time. My sense organs seemed to explode in psychophysical conflict. I heard Connie sigh that it was a custom fit. Actively thrusting my sensitized penis into her vagina, I felt our intermingled lust unlike that of any previous genital copulation. Connie shuddered in orgasmic delight. I knew that her orgasms depended on not only my thrusting.

Several hours later, after my penis had erupted in orgasm, I collapsed in euphoria. Formerly, I'd cuddle with my lustmate after coital activity. Connie didn't elicit those feelings of postcoital affection. I experienced a resistance to that tenderness. My masochized brain said no: I must keep her in the role of dominatrix. Love and lust cannot coexist with Connie. Masochized lust must prevail. Those were the words I was hearing in my brain.

Throughout that week, we copulated daily. Our copulation was oral and anal, as well as genital. With every orgasm of mine, there merged a renewed genital stimulation. I couldn't even have a shower without an inflated penis. Occasionally, Connie would notice my perpetual hard-on, grasp it by the neck, and suck the juice from its swollen head.

I couldn't work or think rationally. Whenever I sensed that Connie pleased me coitally, she'd resume control dominantly. She knew exactly when I needed another masochistic fix, and she would provide it.

Shortly before noon one day, one of my former lovers knocked on my apartment door. Nora had married one of her tricks and moved to New Jersey with him and her son. She returned to Baltimore to visit her sisters and mother. Nora included me during her visit. Connie knew of my previous sexual relationships with Nora and her sisters. In my erotic partnership with Nora, she played the masochistic role and needed domination and spankings. Nora's current partnership was a companionship of convenience.

Nonetheless, Nora invited Connie and me to enjoy her home in New Jersey for a few days. We accepted the invitation. There was a massive flea market near Nora's house in New Jersey, which Connie and I would consider attending while residing at Nora's home, particularly since we possessed twenty X-rated videocassettes that were for sale.

Nora and Connie consorted favorably. Intrapersonally, it thrilled me to mingle with two females who were my bedmates. Unfortunately, Nora's obesity altered her former sexiness, especially concerning my genital arousal. Prior to the lovebond that she and I shared for five years Nora was a stripteaser at the 408 Club on Baltimore's Block. There she displayed herself as an erotic allurement to thousands of the club's customers.

On the day of the New Jersey flea market, my goddess of lust accentuated herself by wearing a skimpy bikini. Her voluptuous figure permeated the sexual brains of the males at the flea market. Connie's blonde hair, protrusive breasts, slender waist, wide hips, and shapely legs diminished the attractiveness of every other female attending that flea market. Thus, Connie's erotic parts precipitated the sale of her X-rated videocassettes within two hours. Every customer questioned the possibility of Connie's appearance in the videos. Admittedly, Connie had misappropriated the videocassettes while employed at a video company.

Connie conveyed the apotheosis of womankind whenever she appeared, especially within my masochized lovemap. While we were sojourning at Nora's home, copulation was spontaneous between Connie and me. I noticed that Nora's son even experienced penile erections when in the proximity of Connie's luring limbs. Also, I sensed an envious attitude from Nora's husband concerning our copulatory activity in their guest room.

Nonetheless, on our return trip to Baltimore, Connie conveyed a diminished desire for coital activity. Coitally, something other than me incited Connie's lust. Yet, I had no concept of its origin—or deleteriousness. Our interpartner paraphilias engendered an ominous reciprocity between us. We were foredoomed.

After returning to my apartment, Connie lost interest in copulation. When she left the apartment, she didn't return until late. When she allowed coitus, it was perfunctory.

In an urgent effort to earn money, we attended another flew market. I attempted to sell my polishing cloths, but failed. After returning, Connie declared what spurred her to lust—robbery! Connie delineated prior robbery episodes with other men, and how those robberies excited her sexually. If I wanted Connie turned on I must do things her way, she explained. Then, purposefully, my empress of lust said, "Robbery with my gun will make me horny again."

Since my rent was due, Connie detailed the means to acquiring money by using her gun. "You want me turned on, don't you?" she asked with a look of menacing confidence. She showed me her pearl-handled gun.

Amazingly, Connie knew how to catch people off guard in the malls. Connie even knew how to identify the mall security. I robbed my first victim under Connie's direction. Performing as my goddess of crime directed, I didn't consider it robbery.

Our first criminally eroticized earnings were spent in an unusual fashion: Connie purchased erotic lingerie. She adorned herself as the goddess of crime. She reveled in her alluring attire, and I reveled in being under her spell masochistically.

Connie adorned herself with a push-up bra, which accentuated her protrusive breasts, a corset, which enhanced the slenderness of her waist, patterned hosiery that embellished her shapely legs, and high-heeled shoes that made her statuesque.

Irrespective of the hour, nothing mattered except that I know and experience unmodified lust with Connie. Resting her back against the corner of my fur-covered couch, Connie gestured for me to kneel at the side of the couch. Parting her vulvar lips, Connie teased me, visuo-erotically. My sexual brain couldn't do anything except gaze at her. Connie's alluring breasts urged my mouth to pant.

"Now you see that robbery is what I need to be turned on, so you must please me. We're going to acquire more money tomorrow. I'll let you look at my pussy and fuck me, but only if you follow my orders," declared Connie, as she stroked my rigid penis.

My mistress of lust tantalized me for several hours. Semen oozed from my engorged penis. While we were in bed together, I tried to sleep, but my aching penis rendered me restless. Connie threatened to strap my penis if I didn't sleep. Thus, my erotic imagery indulged in scenes with Connie whipping, strapping, and beating my buttocks and genitals. Eventually I slept, but I awoke with extreme penile tension.

Awakening before me, Connie arose and prepared coffee, then awakened me to assure my obedience to herself. She stroked my swollen penis with her dainty fingers. She licked my genitals teasingly. Connie frenzied my mind and body with her tongue.

With a rictus of lust, Connie warned, "I'll let you see my pussy tonight. I'll even let you stick your dick in my cunt, but we'd better get what I want today. Now turn over, I'm going to beat your ass."

Turning over as ordered, I trembled in anticipation of her stinging strap. My mistress of pain lashed my helpless buttocks. I cringed in agony until my masochistic metamorphosis occurred. I sensed my flesh being lashed, but the stinging was replaced with euphoria. My masochistic fix desensitized my painful response, and focused my attention on my dominatrix.

Later we drove from mall to mall passing bad checks; Connie's demeanor was audacious. My wicked whore delighted in our spoils. We obtained clothing and jewelry. Connie's capacity for crime intensified. We drove from store to store shoplifting. If she was stopped by mall security, I'd stop them with her gun as instructed.

By the time we arrived home, the car was filled with stolen merchandise. Since our eroticized stealing meant nothing to me, I never considered its worth. Connie's body was my only quest.

Connie portrayed the embodiment of criminalized lust. She enrobed herself with our acquisitions. Connie relished my powerlessness to resist her, as I worshiped her. My testicles ached, for I needed to ejaculate, especially into my wicked whore.

Since that was our first week of eroticized crime, Connie rewarded me with the taste of her titillating flesh. My mistress undressed and reclined on our bed, spreading her shapely thighs. She invited me to lick her labia of lust. My mouth rushed to lap her labial ambrosia. When she was satisfied, I was allowed to penetrate her.

Deeply into Connie's vaginal vise I sunk my protruding penis. It sent waves of sensory stimulus throughout my mind and body. Genitally, the feeling was beyond ordinary stimulation. Reaching behind me, Connie grasped by buttocks. Pulling my body closer, she rubbed her pelvis against mine. Thrusting my penis into her vagina, I was amazed at my undaunted erotic energy. I didn't feel a pending orgasm. It was over an hour of genital reciprocation before my delayed orgasm gushed within her womb.

I slept in orgasmic afterglow until morning. Then we sought another car and stealthily procured different license plates. Our eroticized crime spree continued.

With Connie at my side, we inquired of a car dealer about a car that we might purchase. Taking the car for a test drive, I duplicated the keys. Then, while still test driving the car, we robbed another store. Connie was pleased with me for committing crime. Misappropriating money especially spurred her to lust. I didn't consider the armed robbery a crime; I wasn't even sure that I was awake.

We returned the car to the car dealership. Later that night, we returned with the extra keys, and drove the car off the lot. I followed Connie in our car as she drove it home. Aftger hiding the stolen car, I installed our stolen tags on it.

My mistress of crime lured me into the bedroom. She teased me with her captivating crotch. Gesturing for me to place my rigid penis at the portal of her vagina, Connie grasped my shoulders. Connie planned our malicious work for the next day, as my potent penis begged to enter her. I had no autonomy; my Mephistopheles, my whore of hell, owned me.

That night, our criminalized orgasms were ecstatic. The next morning, Connie ordered me across her lap. Then, with all the force she could summon, she pounded my buttocksd with the wooden paddle. Physically, I'd be capable of rising from Connie's lap, but I couldn't move to resist. My masochized brain needed yet another fix. As Connie's domination pervaded my mind and body, the transformation occurred. Like a wind sweeping across the grass, my pain transformed into a euphoria. It is not the affection of love, nor is it the longing, eagerness, and inclination of lust. It's a protective measure from my vandalized childhood that developed into an entity. Now, instead of protecting me from parental and sisterly torture, it torments me. I'm victimized by myself. Masochistically, I'm totally tractable to Connie, and her paraphilia.

Subsequently, we drove the stolen car out into the country. Stopping at a store with self-service gas pumps, I filled the tank of our car. When I returned from paying for the gasoline, Connie questioned me about the number of people in the store. There was only one teenaged female attendant, I reported.

"Now I'll show you how to rob stores," Connie said threateningly, as she wrapped a blue bandanna around her blonde-haired head and obscured her eyes with stolen sunglasses.

My goddess of crime wasn't nervous, anxious, reluctant, or wary. No, instead she was audacious, intrepid, confident, and aggressive. Connie entered the store menacingly exhibiting her gun. After procuring the store's money, she locked the cashier behind a door within the store. With alacrity she rushed from the store and got into the car.

Connie counted the miscarried money with glee. "I wish that I were a man, so I could do this all the time; people aren't intimidated by women as much as they are by men," said my goddess of crime.

That criminal eroticism wasn't enough. We observed a carryout shop that seemed deserted. Connie moved into the driver's seat and sent me into the carryout. Upon my display of Connie's gun, the cashier panicked and darted toward a rear door. The cash register was full of money. I grasped the currency and change and ran back to Connie, who was waiting in the car with the motor running. Connie verbalized excitement over the abundance of money and accelerated from the parking lot. Skillfully, she drove at speeds of 100 mph and more. Soon we were safely out of that crime zone, but our criminal eroticism had merely begun.

By her own admission, Connie had been committing armed robbery with a male accomplice since the age of thirteen. She knew that I could be led astray by her domination. In order to achieve optimal orgasm with me, she needed to make me a criminal. My erotic high derived from visual contact with Connie's physique, and masochistic imagery of her as dominatrix. There were subliminal clues passed between us that facilitated the development of our eroticized armed robbery. I know that without Connie at my side, I'd never have committed armed robbery. Armed robbery never occurred in my orgasmic fantasies, but it recurred in Connie's erotic imagery. Masochistically, I would have done anything that Connie told me to do. I pleased Connie to keep her with me in order to be spanked again. Lying across Connie's lap was absolute in my paraphilia; I needed my masochistic fixes. Subsequent to our armed robbery episodes, Connie and I would spend hours in orgasms. I was semierect during all armed robbery episodes.

After two weeks, and about twelve armed robberies, Connie and I were unknown to the police. Our reciprocal paraphilias had an uncanny way of surviving within us, although Connie thought that I was outstandingly bad at armed robbery. Fearful of our capture, she utilized my vandalized lust to make me careful.

My mistress and I searched for a place to hold up. She mentioned a likely spot for a hit. As we approached the target, the activity didn't seem real to me. In fact, the criminal fact of committing armed robbery never occurred to me. I was only concerned about being with my mistress. Typically, someone about to commit a felony is nervous, tense, and worries about getting caught. This was not the case with me. I had no scruples about the act of armed robbery or of being shot. In fact, the thoughts never presented themselves in my mind.

I was erotically high, watching her luring limbs. My penis was semierect. I knew only one thing: when we finish this, I'll achieve several orgasms within her vaginal vise. She'll open her legs and let me view her luscious labia. My mind and body will be ecstatic with sexualized energy. There is nothing else.

My mistress stopped near the target. It was a sub shop and it didn't have any customers. I put the gun under my belt. I had to rob to return to her, but I felt solicitous about leaving her.

Walking about one block from the car, I entered the sub shop and ordered a sub from a plump lady. I scanned the shop for my robbery onset. Then I menacingly pointed the gun at the plump lady. She panicked. Suddenly, from around the corner of the store, there appeared a big man with a big gun. Turning swiftly toward the store's door, I ran out and into the night. He followed me quickly with shouts of anger, and his gun. My brain alerted me to only one thing: I must get back to Connie.

Piercing the night, the sound of gunfire riddled the air. Shooting back didn't enter my mind; nothing entered my mind. It was already completely pervaded by my mistress. Interrupting my yearning for her, my pursuer blasted another shot from his gun, which struck a brick wall near me. I ignored it. Soon I'd be with Connie in the car, I thought. Neither my safety, my life, nor the world concerned me. I had to be with Connie for my next orgasmic fix.

My goddess of crime moved her black sedan nearer to me. She pushed the rear door open. I dove onto the floor of the car. Connie slammed the gas pedal to the floor, and the car responded. She warned me to keep down. We heard more gunfire. We traversed a maze of streets and concealed ourselves under the cover of night.

When Connie inquired about my possible injuries, I felt good. All I wanted was to hear her voice and remain in her spell. I desired only to be her slave and lover, and indulge the night in lust.

Connie showed much sympathy toward me. It seemed that she

cared more about my possible wounds than I might have imagined. Since we carried a few thousand dollars from an earlier robbery, we drove to Baltimore's Block. There, my mistress could buy more erotic lingerie and erotic toys.

Reflectively, I considered that I acted much like the dancers who worked on the Block. Most of the strippers pairbond with men who are physically abusive and domineering. They label this attachment love, but love is affectionate. Returning and submitting to an abusive man is not affectionate love, it's distorted love.

My first visit to Baltimore's Block had occurred around my twenty-first birthday. Subsequently, I spent twenty years visiting those clubs. I thrived on the erotic visual stimulation of the stripteasers. I kept mental records on my observations and conversations with all employees on the Block. The bartenders had genital lust for the strippers, but they were totally void of affectionate love for them. Misguidedly, the girls supposed that the longing, eagerness, and inclincation of lust was erotic love.

Tonight, Connie viewed many peep shows. The peep shows were either of lesbian activity or females in bondage. Connie's genital stimulation seemed to elevate by the hour. The visual erotica of magazines, papers, and novels impinged upon my mind. I longed to indulge lustfully with my lustmate. After Connie spent forty dollars on a leather G-string, we drove home. We were high on lust.

While driving home, Connie suggested a variation in our sexual activity. She proposed a bondage game with handcuffs, belt, chains, and phallus. Upon arriving home, Connie removed a cucumber from the refrigerator. She immersed it in hot water and looked at me with a spasm of lust.

We lit candles throughout my apartment and turned off the lamps. Connie put on her enticing apparel. She relished my capitulation, my adoration of her luring physique. I realized I was curious about Connie's interest in bondage, but it didn't matter; I was living only to placate her pudenda of lust.

Wrapping chains around each of Connie's ankles, I secured them to the sides of the bed. Handcuffing her wrists, I affixed the handcuffs to the headboard. Connie instructed me to put rubber bands around her aroused nipples. With her eyes closed, Connie indulged her private realm of lust. With my eyes open, I consumed Connie's restrained body.

Waving my strap salaciously above her, I flicked it upon Connie's pinched nipples. She sighed tensely as I increased the flicking of the strap acorss her increasingly tenderized breasts. Her cunt secreted fluids while I lashed her restrained flesh. Then, interrupting my eroticized whipping, Connie requested the warming cucumber.

I quickly returned to my lustmate with the warmed cucumber. Unfastening the chains at the bottom of the bed, I positioned them so that Connie's legs were forced open widely. I gazed at Connie's cunt as though life had nothing else to offer.

Pressing the tip of the large cucumber into the labial opening, I wedged it into Connie's vagina. She tensed from the cucumber's intrustion, but the deeper it dug, the more she welcomed it. Although restrained, she controlled our fantasy-inspired scenario.

I remembered the nights with another girl who had performed masochistically with me. She was the masochist to my sadist. For the first year of our lustbond, I chained her to our bed nightly. She reveled in the eroticized bondage. I frequently bound her body with her buttocks elevated. I beat her rump with a paddle and a strap. Sometimes I dripped candle wax on her helpless behind.

Eventually, the sadomasochism reached a point of revulsion. I chewed her nipples and she urged me to chew to draw blood. That urging failed, for I couldn't do it. Eventually I couldn't cope with her masochism at all.

Nonetheless, here I am in another sadomasochistic lustbond. While Connie squeezed her embedded cucumber, I inundated her flesh with my mouth, lips, and tongue. I longed to dislodge the cucumber and insert my panting penis.

Connie urged me to insert my oozing penis into her gaping mouth. Straddling her head with my knees, I introduced my eager penis to her receptive mouth and tongue. My state of masochistic arousal needed sensual stimulation. Not ordinary stimulation, however. I asked Connie to bite the skin of my overaroused penis. I slid my rigid cock along the rows of Connie's teeth. She chewed and bit my penis. My head began to frenzy. Thrusting to the throat's portal and withdrawing, my penis elevated my senses into another realm.

Finally, Connie sucked the sperm from my erupting penis—but its engorgement didn't diminish. Removing the phallic cucumber, I entered Connie's vagina of lust with my overpotent penis. It seemed as though every sense organ within my body urged me to a second penile climax. Connie's quim was grasping, sliding, and rotating on my brawny penis, varying the rhythm, speed, and intensity. Perspiration dripped from my skin onto Connie's own perspiring flesh. No words were uttered, no endearments, only engulfing movements.

I'll never know what mentally criminal scenario permeated Connie's vandalized lovemap to facilitate her orgasms, but my own orgasm spurted with images of Connie's domination of me.

Connie needed another orgasmic fix within two days. My genital tension was really never assuaged. Connie planned another day of eroticized crime. This time we disguised ourselves. After stealing the items needed to alter our appearance, we prepared for our illicit masquerade.

Once a robbery target was picked, Connie would enter the place to locate the doors and count the people. Then Connie would hand me her gun to perpetrate the robbery. By the end of that day Connie and I had robbed four establishments. All the while, I experienced only genital lust toward my lustmate.

Feeling the force of her own paraphilic stimulation, Connie suggested that we find a video motel. We purchased alcohol and pot before we lodged at the X-rated motel. Connie dressed in her erotic lingerie, and I filled the ice bucket. Strangely, Connie needed to enrobe herself in alluring apparel. Although I enjoyed the enhancement of her physique in the lingerie, my sexual brain never imaged her that way.

Connie forked her luring thighs while leaning against the headboard and watching an X-rated video. I reclined in front of her to peer between her thighs. Entranced by her voracious vulva. I became oblivious to anything else. While Connie stared at X-rated movies, I performed cunnilingus on her by the hour. When her pampered pudenda was ready for penetration, I mounted her pelvis and launched my penis deep within her.

Several days later, Connie semed placid. So far, we'd perpetrated two dozen armed robberies, all erotically inspired. I drove to fill the gas tank. While driving that day, Connie had something interesting to say.

"I seem to have lost the desire for robbery. I've felt like this before. The feeling for robbery comes and goes. I don't understand it, but we'll quit for a while," she said, gazing out the car window.

Unfortunately, that meant Connie wouldn't be horny anymore. For the next week, she seemed disoriented. She would leave the apartment and return late. My entire existence was in a turmoil of frenzied lust. I couldn't leave the apartment, nor could I eat with enjoyment. My masochism still cried out for another satiation.

Then, one night, when Connie was absent, my masochized brain urged me to spank myself. Irrespective of how my orgasm was achieved, the intense stimulation of spanking transports me into another realm. To please Connie, and arouse her genitally, I wondered if I could commit armed robbery by myself. I couldn't.

Since we spent the misappropriated money as quickly as we acquired it, I tried to earn money legally. But I remained distracted. I wished that I could die, for the images of my brain tormented me. But I couldn't even pull the trigger on Connie's gun to end my masochistic torture.

Reflectively, I observed that Connie exhibited another personality when she left the apartment. She typically portrayed the quintessence of femininity and allurement, but when she went out without me she'd wear black boots, jeans, a studded leather jacket, studded wristbands, a T-shirt, and a blue bandanna. With her long blonde hair, shapeley thights, slender waist, wide hips, and beautiful face, Connie was strikingly erotic. Although her apparel appeared masculinized, her demeanor was passively female. Conversely, feminine apparel evoked her nature as the dominatrix and goddess of crime. Had I met Connie in her masculinized attire, my masochism would not have been evoked.

However, I had met Connie when she was wearing feminized attire. Thus, I viewed her as my dominatrix whether she wanted that role or not. Connie was cast into a role without her consent, just as my sexual brain cast her into that role without my consent. The only way that I imaged myself with Connie was draped across her thighs being spanked. My eroticized brain longed for the stimulus of looking at her viewable vulva, instead of penetrating it with my erect penis. With almost any other women, I would seek genital reciprocity. Paraphilias are not only ineffaceable, they're selfish, for they demand their own expression irrespective of the person they possess or inhabit.

With Connie and myself, the self is divided. Our experience is like that of Dr. Jekyll and Mr. Hyde. Similar to Dr. Jekyll, I am a professional salesman and marketing manager. Yet, as Mr. Hyde, I am a masochist and armed robber. Perhaps Dr. Jekyll had a predisposition to emerge like the monster Mr. Hyde, which is why he discovered the formula to induce that metamorphosis. Perhaps we are all predisposed to another self, but some of us find the inducement to an altered self, and some of us do not. Contrary to the dictionary definition of masochism, I do not find pleasure in masochistic behavior of inflicted pain. I find it terrifying, inconvenient, dangerous, uncomfortable, and addictive. My masochized high is addictive, not pleasurable.

My obsequiousness with Connie sickened me and sometimes her. One night, Connie grew weary of my masochized personality. She ordered me into the bedroom and handcuffed my hands behind my back. My penis was extended and rigid. Connie lashed my erection until it appeared like a red sore. Welts covered my skin. My masochized brain thrived on the pain inflicted. My penis oozed steadily. Inexplicably, I didn't want Connie to cease beating my penis. Then she made me lie on my stomach and commenced pounding my buttocks with her wooden paddle. When she was satisfied with her punishment, she left the bedroom with my wrists still handcuffed. She kept me restrained until morning. My masochized stimulation prevailed.

Our money supply was deficient. Connie was reluctant to play the role of hooker to earn money. We actually prowled with that intention a few nights. Connie recalled, and conveyed to me, situations whereby she'd lure a potential customer into a seculuded area, then her accomplice would bludgeon him. Insouciently they would take his money and valuables and leave him victimized.

Our eroticized robbery spree had extended over Baltimore City, Baltimore County, and Ann Arundal County. Now we planned to leave the state with more armed robbery in our paraphilic minds. Connie's mother lived in Delaware, so that was our aim. During the drive, Connie smoked pot and held my hand. She presided over me like my mother. She would display affection, then without notice be cruel both verbally and physically. My mother would say, "I love you," then she would scream, "I hate you." Unfortunately, I was addicted to that conflict.

Tractably, I served Connie. I'd light her cigarettes, buy her sodas or coffee, and act like an uxorious husband. Upon arriving at her mother's home, Connie intensified her affection toward me. With most women, I would relish that display of affection, but not with Connie. Curiously, Connie bantered with her mother as though they were merely friends. Her mother accepted me and strived to please me while residing in her home.

That first night at her mother's house, we indulged in much loveplay and genital coupling. Connie's lust was accommodating. I kissed every inch of Connie's flesh fervently. I sucked at Connie's delicious breasts. When Connie parted her pretty thighs, I licked, lapped, and sucked her luscious labia. Her vaginal juice overwhelmed my senses.

Delightfully, I penetrated Connie's snugly fitting vagina. Connie drew her knees back to her shoulders and compassionately suggested that I thrust my penis until I was exhausted. I hugged Connie while thrusting into her receptive vessel of lust. Curiously, Connie embraced me as though she knew that I suffered mentally. Then, orgasmically we feel asleep.

During the next delightful day, we copulated in the shower and on the couch. Connie displayed much affectionate love, but I was unable to dislodge her dominatrix demeanor from my imagery. Also, Connie reiterated her reluctance to continue armed robbery. Connie's mixed sexuality perplexed and frustrated me. Yet, while residing at her mother's house, our sexual activity was frequent and almost fulfilling.

We departed Connie's mother's home and Delaware without committing crime. Connie's paraphilia subsided, but my masochism still raged within my mind. Our paraphilias were no longer reciprocal. I sensed something ominous, but I couldn't identify it.

Upon arriving in Balitmore, back at my apartment, Connie dressed in her masculinized attire. I returned to alcohol as my coping mechanism. Our verbal discourse was bitter and hostile. Connie refused to play the role of dominatrix anymore. She was disinclined to indulge sexually with me. Then, self-destruction took over.

On August 30, 1984, Connie left my apartment for the last time. She bought and smoked two cans of "greens." Her mind, like mine, was in turmoil. She went to a police station and turned us in.

3

The Victim Is the Accused
Enlightenment of Paraphilic Ignorance

The humidity and heat permeated my cozy apartment that foreboding August. Sitting, standing, or walking failed to relieve my lovesickness and despair. An obsessive yearning to be near Connie haunted my masochized mind and body.

Intermittently I questioned the existence of my reputed power of choice. I didn't choose to be genitally aroused by replica images of my mother and sister, who had dominated me. It just happened. I didn't choose to spend my earnings in pursuit of paraphilic lust, but I did it. I would choose to escape this vile vise that is destroying me, but it holds me in its grip. If I had had a choice I wouldn't be here. If there were a god of caring, that god would choose to rescue me.

Several hours after midnight, I attempted to sleep, but Connie's physical absence prevented it. My imagery portrayed her face, demeanor, and voluptuous physique. My imagery staged me kneeling in front of her luring vulva. Masochistically, I longed to be draped across her thighs while being spanked to an orgasm.

An undetermined amount of time lapsed. Then noises at my door alarmed me. Anticipating the arrival of my mistress, I arose to greet her. Suddenly and intrusively, four pistols and two shotguns threatened me. I faced the menacing police and their weapons with total apathy. With Connie's little derringer that didn't fire, what kind of resistance could I have put up? I watched myself being handcuffed.

The police destroyed and ransacked my apartment for evidence, but didn't observe what was in full view. There were chains attached to the four corners of the bed. My own handcuffs were hanging on the bedroom doorknob. A wooden paddle and strap with which my mistress spanked and strapped me were under the couch. Connie's erotic lingerie added up to at least fifty outfits.

The terroristic police treated me as guilty, not as innocent until proven guilty, and without a reasonable doubt. They didn't read me my constitutional rights. They refused to permit me a phone call. I was cruelly escorted to a patrol car. This was my first criminal act. I felt betrayed.

Before the police break-in, I had ingested several pills of Dalmane, but no sleeping pills would allow me to sleep at the police station that night. I could think only of Connie.

Sometime during the next day, two detectives conferred with me. Sadly, I discovered that Connie had reported us to the police. They had no evidence of our mutual involvement in armed robbery until Connie had revealed it. It was in the script of Connie's own paraphilia to report us, blaming me. Without hesitation, I confessed to my part in the commission of armed robbery. I even signed a confession. Mostly, I yearned for death. Only death would stop my paraphilia of masochism. Like most people who are prone to suicide, I sought to destroy not the self, but the tormentor within the self. Unfortunately, I had no legal right to die, only to suffer.

Inexplicably, Connie's betrayal and my arrest halted my erotic and paraphilic imagery. My genitalia didn't swell anymore. I was perplexed about my lack of erotic interest, but I felt quite relieved. Genital arousal and accompanying erotic imagery disappeared for exactly one year following my incarceration.

After my bail hearing, I was transported to the Baltimore City Jail. My bail was forty times that of Connie's bail. Since her bail amounted to only $10,000, Connie was out of jail shortly thereafter.

A jail is populated with sexually distorted inmates, but the staff knows little about their paraphilias. I could easily see why there is so much recidivism. At the Baltimore City Jail, an inmate spends every hour of the day competing with other inmates and institutional officers. There is no opportunity for improvement. Moreover, every inmate is stigmatized as guilty even before trial.

I couldn't afford an attorney. So the state provided me with a public defender, then another, and another. The third one accepted my defense of erotomania. Since I was just learning about paraphilia, I didn't use that word. Now I wish I had.

At my arraignment, my lawyer entered a plea of not guilty by reason of insanity, due to erotomania. I'm told I was the first person in the state to have used that defense. However, that was merely a mitigative defense, for I know what I did with Connie, but not why I did it.

Subsequently, the state's forensic specialists interrogated and tested me. On the inkblot test, I perceived female images in every inkblot. That was too close to being virtually unheard of. The state denied the validity of my inkblot associations. In fact, I had perceived nothing but female forms in those inkblots.

A videotaping was scheduled for my unprecedented defense. However, instead of seeking truth, the state's forensic experts strived to discredit my account of erotomania. For example, after I said that Connie carried her own gun, the state's doctor replied that all the prostitutes he knew carried guns. I questioned that, for I've hired two hundred prostitutes, or more, and only a few of them carried a gun. Mostly they were sweet girls. When I stated that the gunshots didn't disturb me, they didn't believe that either. But that's the way it happened.

For one of my psychological tests, I was asked to draw a picture of a person. Now, I can't even draw a straight line, but I'm asked to draw a person. I attempted to cooperate, but the drawing was feeble. Naturally, I attempted to draw a female, for I rarely imagine any other species. In the drawing, the arms were behind the female figure. Art is not my forte. However, because I didn't draw the hands of the female, it was inferred by the state's psychologist that I had a castration complex. To me, that sounded absurd.

Further interrogation continued at Clifton T. Perkins, the prison hospital for the criminally insane. My aim was to get this thing over with, for C. T. Perkins was worse than the Baltimore City Jail. During another session of psychological testing, the state's psychologist asked questions that seemed irrelevant. Well, since I longed to get out of Perkins, I brought her back to the subject. Consequently, when the psychologist testified in court, that was held against me.

At no time during any interrogative proceedings did anyone examine my masochistic partnership with Connie. Nor did they ever ask

Connie so far as I know, whether she had played the role of my dominatrix and spanked me.

After being returned to the Baltimore City Jail, I awaited my first trial, which finally took place seven months after I'd been arrested. While confined at the jail, I discovered some important things. In short, the only way for an inmate to survive is to lie, cheat, and steal. Goodness is a weakness, badness is a virtue, and covert retaliation is encouraged by the staff. All inmates manifest a distortion of their masculine gender identity. Their manhood is based upon the cultural ideals and social advertising they have encountered. The result: distortion.

Finally, my trial date arrived. I was transported to the county courthouse in Towson, but in the afternoon instead of the morning. At the end of my first of ten days in court, the judge ordered my detention at the Baltimore County Detention Center. Because of the judge's change of my confinenent, I lost all of the legal material I had worked on for seven months. That included my copy of *Love and Lovesickness* and my clothing. My opinion is that the court wanted to separate me from my defense material.

The next day was jury selection. The state's prosecutor didn't like my counsel or me. She made sure that no jury members were sympathetic to my defense. Moreover, she didn't allow any young females to sit on the jury, although that would have made it more a jury of my peers. After all, my entire life had been in proximity of young women, and my crimes were committed with a female.

Finally, my jury consisted of what I considered twelve nonorgasmic, hypophilic, erotically apathetic, inert, and unworldly jurors. Of course, that suited my androgynous prosecutor quite well.

During my trial in Towson, any persons entering the courtroom were warned of my trial's sexualized content. A reporter sat in the courtroom, but the subsequent reporting in the *Sun* paper was quite inaccurate. Of course, I was not permitted to give the reporters any information.

Daily I strove to speak between the prosecutor's objections. The problem with the jury, prosecutor, and judge amounted to ignorance of paraphilia or any other sexual disorder. Since a grown man doesn't typically drape himself across the lap of his young girlfriend, to be spanked to an orgasm, I had to be giving false information. In vain did I discard my idealized manliness to tell the truth about my paraphilic lust affair with Connie.

Ideally, the courts should detect all paraphilic defendants, and cease vulgarizing the words sex and lust. After all, my activities with Connie were a result of a distorted lust and an impaired love, not sex. While waiting for trial, I had learned that there are forty-odd paraphilias, many of which are harmful, a few harmless. Some paraphilias pose a malignant threat to society, especially to women and children. Furthermore, young children living with a paraphilic parent can become predisposed to developing as a paraphile. Paraphiles cannot be cured but they can be helped. However, prison will not help.

Contrary to the assertions of the state's prosecutor, I didn't seek reprieve, forgiveness, or exoneration. Something inhabited me, making me behave contrary to social and personal standards. I needed the help that the sexual disorders clinic at The Johns Hopkins Hospital could have provided me. My sickness or disorder required treatment, not condemnation and imprisonment. Actually, the prison environment disposes the paraphile for more paraphilic behavior through its rehearsal in fantasy. After all, a paraphile isn't born with a paraphilia. Family members and other unknown forces predispose a child to a paraphilia. Then, from its own ignorance, society forces the paraphile into covert activity.

The subject of alcohol was introduced into the case because I had written about my consumption of alcohol in my diary. However, no one considered the fact that I drank alcohol as a coping strategy. Perhaps most, if not all, alcoholic men and women drink alcohol as a coping strategy. Paraphilias are psychophysically tormenting. For me alcohol was self-medication, not a way to get high.

My high was my own orgasm. One of the state's doctors read in my diary that I paid $1.99 for Coke. Then he erroneously inferred that I bought and injected cocaine. The fool! There isn't any amount of cocaine that sells for $1.99. Only Coca-Cola is that price. In any case, my masochistic orgasm exceeded the high of any drug.

I was found guilty. So also was Connie in another courtroom. Imagery of Connie had faded from my mind, and I still didn't experience penile lust over any female image.

In court I had a problem with legal jargon, which kept me from defending myself properly. As I studied paraphilic sexology, a whole new language emerged. As in the ordinary person, my knowledge of my innermost sexuality was quite limited. Indeed, the English language doesn't even carry a respectable vernacular word for intergenital activity, or a reciprocal verb for it.

For example, when one of the state's psychologists questioned me, I commented that I had to have an orgasm every day. He retorted with, "Lots of people have an orgasm every day." Well, that wasn't exactly what I meant to say. In short, if I didn't ejaculate daily, my body refused to function properly until I did achieve an orgasm. However, it is not merely an orgasm, for a specified scenario must accompany that orgasm. If my actual world would match my mental world, then my orgasm would occur. I had trouble just masturbating.

I wrote letters to Connie, which might incite her to play dominatrix by mail. Words, written or voiced, are an impetus to lust, and to the manifestation of lust, which is genital arousal. However, Connie did not reply with words to spur my lust, genital arousal, or orgasm. Our armed robbery orgasms were gone forever.

Connie and I were consigned from Baltimore County to the State Division of Corrections. However, that was not the end of our criminal charges. We still had charges of armed robbery to face in Anne Arundel County.

The erotica of former inmates covered the walls of my cell at the prison, but my erotic brain and genitals were still inactive. I'd sit on my bunk and wonder why the erotica didn't rouse me to lust. Masochism wasn't alone the incitement to my lust, I hoped. I thought that the erotica on my walls might substitute for my sadomasochism. It wouldn't. Only after many more months of study would I begin to understand which type of erotica would or would not arouse me to lustfulness.

I longed to be orgasmic again. Can you believe that? I'm facing ten years of incarceration, and I still have a longing for genital arousal, especially arousal induced by Connie. Although I hated being a masochist, I would have sacrificed another year of being in prison just to be spanked to ecstasy. Yet, Connie would never again induce such an orgasmic ecstasy. I'm not addicted to my sexual disorder; it *inhabits* me. My paraphilia still lurked within my mind, albeit inactively.

Inexplicably, along with my inactive paraphilia, my bipolar, manic-depressive up and down moods were also inactive. My brain functioned better during this period than at any former time in my life.

Connie and I were eventually ordered to court in Anne Arundel County. Since we were both confined in Jessup, Maryland, we were escorted to court in Annapolis in the same vehicle. I rode in the van from the House of Correction to the Maryland Correctional Institute for Women. I watched Connie walk in handcuffs and shackles toward the van. Then, and for the first time in ten months, I sat in tactual and vocal proximity to my former dominatrix. It was amusing for both of us, for we had formerly chained each other in the course of achieving our armed robbery orgasms. In fact, I still carried my handcuff key.

Connie is a beautiful blonde by even the most exacting standards. Even so, I didn't feel an erotic or paraphilic inclination toward her, and I was seated right next to her. I asked myself, "What really makes the penis swell, and why does it swell more with one girl than another girl?" Unfortunately, I had begun the sacrifice of fifteen years of my life for a woman who didn't arouse my lust anymore. During the eroticized robberies, and the ensuing orgasms, I never, even once, thought about ending up in prison.

In the van, we conversed mostly about the difference between the women's and men's prisons. Connie revealed to me her lesbian affair with another female inmate. In fact, she stated, she was glad that she was in prison, for she was in lesbian love.

In the Ann Arundel County Court, we received concurrent sentences. When I told the court that Connie spanked me, there was absolute silence. I continued with, "I would have followed her into hell, for I had to be spanked again by my dominatrix." I set a precedent, then.

While traveling with Connie on another court occasion, she revealed some interesting history about herself. She'd been ingesting, inhaling, and injecting mind-altering drugs since the age of thirteen. Being in prison had released her from the availability of those mind-altering coping strategies. Never before, she said, had she felt so good.

I was not the only man she had sent to prison, but this was the first time she herself had been incarcerated. Why had she indulged in mind-altering drugs? It was her own sexual disorder, which I now know is hybristophilia—in short, being genitally and erotically aroused by a criminal partner. In my case, she directed me, her capitulatory slave, into criminal acts, thereby fulfilling the requirements of her own paraphilia. Just as I had used alcohol to cope with my paraphilia, Connie had used psychotropic drugs to cope with hers.

Connie agreed with me about feeling like Dr. Jekyll and Ms. Hyde. "I can't hurt you now, but it was easy to spank you and make you do what I wanted then," she disclosed. I am amazed at how reciprocal our respective paraphilias are.

When the cell door closed behind me, I realized that the doors of the Division of Correction wouldn't open for me again for at least seven years. Within my cell, I charted a course for my future years of incarceration. I needed a new career, and I was determined to know all that was possible to know about paraphilias and other sexual disorders.

In preparation for a new career, I wrote to a friend asking him to send me a typewriter. With little knowledge of professional writing, and no knowledge of typewriting, I planned to become a writer. At that time, I was unaware that the Division of Correction resists the self-improvement of inmates, albeit covertly. Unless an inmate participates in an institutional program, the institution won't recognize the effort. That's an unspoken rule.

Discovering sexology was the second part of my plan. Specific mental imagery or fictive imagery accompanied every episode of my masochistic orgasms. Therefore, I set out to examine the imagery and ideation of my brain and mind. I knew that I needed guidance from the one and only expert in the field: Dr. John Money. I sent him a letter revealing my plan to examine the erotic and nonerotic fantasies pervading my mind. He replied with encouraging interest. My introspection commenced and has continued throughout my incarceration. I determined to memorize and know the meaning of each and every paraphilia.

On the anniversary of my first year of confinement my genital arousal and erotic imagery were still inactive. That amazed me. I was delighted, but I missed orgasmic stimulation. I also longed for the feminine voice, the female demeanor, and the feminine physique. I found it quite difficult living in proximity to foul men who do nothing but degrade femininity in everything they do or say.

It was September 1985. I walked along my tier. Suddenly, my eye glanced at an erotic pictorial in one of the cells on my tier. That female image reached right into my brain's lovemap. In the same second my genitals experienced an engorgement. Activation of my eroticized fantasy or imagery had recrudesced, but without my consent.

Significantly, the pictorial I observed displayed a girl's buttocks. The exact position and form of her buttocks reciprocated an imprint within my brain's lovemap. It suggested imagery, ideation, and orgasms. In accordance with my introspecting I recorded all future scenarios that accompanied my orgasms. At the outset, my orgasms were four and five per day. Between orgasms my typewriter recorded the mental scenes, performers, and activity.

Subsequently, I mailed copies of my fictive imagery to Dr. Money. With his expert guidance, I began to comprehend what the eroticized imagery meant. The interconnections of erotic fantasies explained why my former life led me to Connie and to prison. That was just the beginning.

4

The Paraphilic Fugue

Paraphilia Manifested

Although I estimate that I've earned in excess of one million dollars, all told, I don't have a penny remaining of it. There are days I've awakened to, then somehow lost. There are times when, driving my car to one destination, I'd find myself driving in the wrong direction. While I had a wife and a mistress, I still paid another girl to show me her vulva. Mysteriously, I found myself doing things I would never normally choose to do. Many times, for example, I've driven off the road to achieve an orgasm, but without conscious consent. I've had an eviction notice in my pocket, but instead of paying my overdue rent, I'd pay to look at a specific girl. My coital activities have never been deficient, so I don't do these things out of desperation, loneliness, or horniness. I've driven for five hours to pick up a girl, then paid her five hundred dollars, all just view her vulva.

People have asked me this question for years: "Why, when you're so intelligent, do you do such dumb things?" Well, it's called the paraphilic fugue. It occurs just like Mr. Hyde emerging from Dr. Jekyll. It is triggered by different things and different people. It doesn't care about my health or safety. It doesn't respect those within its path. It can kill, brutalize, and rape. Yes, it might even make one pull the trigger on oneself, and over nothing more than masochism unfulfilled.

In the following examples, I've written about my experiences with the paraphilic fugue. It may seem unbelievable, but it's all true.

I was married and living in Baltimore. Receiving my first American Express Card delighted me. After I arrived home, I couldn't wait to leave. If I said to my wife, Karen, that I was horny, she would lead me to the bedroom. However, my eroticized brain needed another type of stimulation or high. If I had had a choice, I would have stayed home with my wife. Instead I gave her some excuse to leave, and I departed.

My car seemed to know the way to Baltimore's Block, where my brain, through my eyes, would locate a particular type of female. I would want to go home, but I couldn't. After several beers in various clubs, my brain would locate the right girl. My genital arousal under the aegis of the paraphilic fugue was different than ordinary genital arousal. It was an irrepressible force inducing me to achieve an orgasm according to a specific scenario.

She danced on stage. Her name was Cindy. Cindy's body was a match to my ephebophilic lovemap. Seeing her elevated the entrancement of my lust for viewing the pudenda of young girls. I bought a few bottles of champagne for Cindy. Somehow, I moved the conversation to seeing her vulva in private. She agreed since I offered her a hundred dollars, and I had already spent a hundred on her. Part of my paraphilia is chrematistophilia, a love of transacting money for sex.

The Villa Nova bar has seats concealed toward the rear of the club. Cindy and I occupied one of those seats. She tugged her bikini panties down her shapely legs. Spreading her thighs, I gazed at her delicious vulva. Moreover, I stared at her vulva as though something held me there. My engorged penis oozed fluid, but I hadn't touched it. Nonetheless, there was a reciprocal match between my vandalized lovemap and her delectable vulva.

The eager bartender sought more money for having more time with her. Again, I handed him my credit card. I felt inclined to view her tantalizing crotch until my credit limit was reached. Cindy might view her crotch in a mirror, but she wouldn't get the high that I would. Dozens of men might seek to gaze at her breasts or buttocks, but still not experience genital lust like mine. Eventually, I spent six hundred dollars with Cindy, but I never touched her.

My brain was inhabited by Cindy's shapely thighs and vulva. My wife was waiting for me when I arrived home. We went to bed. Our coital activities went on for several hours. I achieved many orgasms, but the impetus to lust wasn't my wife. The images within my vandalized lovemap were of the stripteaser, and those images of her vulva sustained my genital arousal.

The sadomasochism that eventually led me to escort Connie into armed robbery existed in a state of paraphilic fugue. The above scene with Cindy was the same, a paraphilic fugue, but with a different expression.

It was Chicago 1974. I was living there with Nora. Coitally I was content, but another genital stimulus was unsatisfied. Cryptically, I started to drive to where I'd find the strip clubs, which was on Rush Street. Now I am driving without impairment, but I 'm not doing what I really want to do. The urging to view the vulva is without option. My brain needs to thrive on naked ladies.

Nora herself was a stripper. If I went home and told her to dance for me, she would do it. I sanctified my lust for her by living with her, as though we were married. I didn't know about the split of love from lust, then.

I had three hundred dollars in my pocket, which I needed for Nora and me. Yet, I kept driving toward Rush Street. I couldn't turn my car around and go home. Actually, I wanted to be home and hug my lover. Alas, my paraphilia overrode every other interest of mine. Whatever the sacrifice, it would be satisfied.

Arriving near the massage parlors and strip clubs, I was tense and genitally aroused. While strolling along Rush Street, I saw a massage parlor. It incited the interest of my erotic brain. Ambivalently, I entered the massage parlor in quest of that specific female form that would induce optimal genital stimulation. There was a young lady there whose face and physique evoked my interest. My money meant nothing more to me than to facilitate her tantalizing of me.

Alluringly, she posed for me, exhibiting her buttocks, anus, and vulvar cleft. Staring at her erotic parts was like ambrosia to my paraphilic brain. There was a disinclination to touch her, for my stimulation was visual, not tactual. But, viewing her was merely an appetizer. I departed in quest of another stimulus.

Across the street, I entered a strip club. The stripteaser reciprocated the images of my lovemap. After she danced, I bought a drink for her. Then she sat on my lap. I explained some of my lustfulness to her, for she wanted to know why I was there so early in the day.

With a confused look, she asked, "Why doesn't making love work?" I couldn't reply, for I didn't understand. The question disturbed me, so I ran out of the club before I cried. However, I couldn't return home until I experienced intense orgasmic stimulation.

Later I entered another lounge with stripteasers. I observed a female image that matched the image of my erotic brain. The girl wore a silk dress that clung to her proportionally perfect breasts, waist, hips, and thighs. My penis swelled.

Her voice mesmerized me. My masochistic brain had located my dominatrix type. I was oblivious to everything around me, and all other aspects of my life. My genital arousal was intense. I was impaired from seeing her as anything other than a dominatrix.

We sat in a corner where the light didn't intrude. I spoke with her about my sexual disorder. I described my live-in lover. I complained about my masochistic feelings, which recurred episodically. Understandingly, she said that she'd been hired by many men who needed to be dominated and spanked. Within my trouser leg, my organ of lust was on the verge of ejaculation, but I hadn't touched it.

My dominatrix's stand-in talked with me, as though she were my goddess of lust. We bandied words that confected a masochistic scenario. My whole organism lingered with her ecstatically. The longing to sense the sting of a paddle was frustrating. She could have whipped my buttocks until death consumed me, yet I would have died in ecstasy. Temporarily, my vandalized lovemap quenched its paraphilic lust, but only until another day.

While driving home, I was intensely stimulated. I was caught speeding, but I had no knowledge of my speed at the time. Although I occupied the driver's seat, my brain replayed the night's events. When I arrived home, my absence had made Nora cry, but I couldn't help it. The paraphilic fugue isn't respectful of persons.

I was a self-employed traveling salesman. One week, I worked in and around a small town called Kittening, Pennsylvania. After work one day, I felt an urging for genital stimulation. The town had little to offer in erotica, but I found an adult book store.

Upon entering the book store, my eyes scanned the shelves of magazines and novels. I discovered provocative erotica. I know that it is my type of erotica, for a surge of blood will rush into my penis. Then I felt myself overpowered with a yearning to experience orgasms.

Fortunately, my hotel was only a mile from the book store. Urgently I returned to view the erotica I had purchased, and to achieve orgasm.

One female image among all the others was prepotent. It was of a brunette squatting with a dress, but without panties. Her vulvar cleft and labia aroused me genitally. Subsequently, her salacious image dominated my mental stage. With that impetus to lust, I achieved many orgasms before morning, but her lusty image would not leave me.

My independence and sense of responsibility disposed me to resume my work as a salesman. Nonetheless, I experienced an inquietude while departing for work. When I began driving, something impaired my ability to drive. Then I experienced a decrease in my psychophysical energy. It was the paraphilic fugue, even though I didn't know it by name at that time.

Suddenly, I lost my volition and physical energy. I couldn't press the pedal of my car with my foot. My hands lost their grip of the steering wheel. My eyes ceased to focus, my eyelids closed involuntarily. Consequently, I drove onto the shoulder of the road and stopped the car. Flopping onto the seat of the passenger's side of the car, I was in a paralysis of confusion. I felt a strange, intense urge to be orgasmic. I wondered why this had happened. I was permeated by an irresistible force to return to my hotel. I could not sit up. I strained myself and got behind the wheel. With diminished capacity, I started the car and drove back to my hotel.

Upon arriving at the hotel, I was weak and found it difficult to open the door. Yet, direly pervading my mind and body was the compulsion to achieve orgasms, and there was no weakness in genital arousal. Mentally, the image of the girl from the previous night's pictorial with her vulvar cleft showing inhabited my mind's eye .

My erection's urging to ejaculate overrode even my efforts to take my suit off. After ejaculating twice, I found relief from the intense orgasmic inclination. Exhaustion overcame me, and I passed out. Several hours later, when I awoke, it was with a continued spurring to ejaculate. Finally, after many orgasms, I slept.

The next day I worked, but not without a reissue of that girl's vulvar cleft intermittently on my mental screen. The female crutch has always elicited my obedient attention.

Another episode of paraphilic fugue occurred while I was driving near King of Prussia, Pennsylvania. I needed to earn much money, which meant that sales must be abundant that day. I was spending about a thousand dollars per month on my mistress, Dawn. While driving, I drank several cups of coffee. There was no prelude to what was about to happen when, suddenly, I felt as though something had drained the energy out of my mind and body, even though I had slept quite well the previous night. Driving to my destination couldn't be stopped now. I was sixty miles from home. Then, a tingling in my genitals prodded me. I wanted to ignore this penile prodding, for I yearned to earn. Soon my legs twitched involuntarily. My penis swelled and oozed. My driving was impaired. I couldn't focus on the road. My reflexes slowed to a standstill. Finally, my eyes refused to remain open. Although I couldn't define it, I knew something strange was happening.

A gush of erotic imagery inhabited me mentally. At first, it was of female parts. Then they became woven into a scene. My genitals and brain seemed to have a direct connection. The urge to stop and ejaculate dominated me. I screamed in resistance, but to no avail. If only there had been someone to turn to!

On the left side of the road, there was an old building. I drove behind the building and rested my tormented head on the steering wheel. All I could imagine were the pear-shaped buttocks of several girls. My engorged penis released its vital fluid.

It was a Sunday night. I departed Baltimore for Pittsburgh. It would be a six-hour drive, at least. My aim was to earn about $2,000. While driving, I mused over many sales situations. By the time I reached Breezewood, Pennsylvania, I had a premonitory warning of a paraphilic fugue. The urging for orgasm felt similar to the urge to urinate, but I didn't need to urinate. Then the imagery of my mental screen eroticized. This time the images were masochized. They won center stage. Once it starts, my paraphilic imagery is impossible to dislocate.

My penile erection maintained its rigidity over the next three hours of driving, always with paraphilic imagery, of course. My room was reserved and waiting for me when I arrived in Pittsburgh. I entered my room, feeling an urgency to ejaculate. Usually, I can diminish my orgasmic intensity through masturbation, but not this time. Even after I achieved an enrapturing orgasm, I longed for another orgasm, and another.

Monday morning, I couldn't arise. My paraphilic imagery and urging for ejaculatory orgasm had intensified instead of diminishing. Since I could afford a day off, I stayed in bed with my erect penis. The more orgasms I achieved, the more I yearned for. My brain thrived on its masochized imagery and ideation. My seminal fluid didn't diminish after each ejaculation, which was unusual.

Tuesday morning I felt paralyzed with eroticized imagery and ideation. I hadn't eaten in twenty-four hours. Since much of my orgasmic imagery was of Dawn, my mistress in Baltimore, I phoned her, but she didn't answer. I supposed that I should eat food, but I wasn't hungry. Taking a walk, I found the hotel bar. I drank one beer, then returned to my room. Stepping into my room, I realized that I hadn't turned the televison on, which is what I normally would have done. My mind was staged with Dawn's physique and visage. I phoned her again. Well, my mistress was preoccupied, especially since I was expected to be out of town that week. Even on the telephone, Dawn swelled my genitalia.

Wednesday morning, I sensed an urgency to do something. I drove in search of those wonderful girls who charge for sexualized activity. Usually, if I can reenact the intrusive imagery, words, and scenario, I'll find relief. Finding a young female to play the role of a dominatrix is rarely accomplished. Most women are inured to the male, and erroneously suppose that he should dominate. However, I did arrange an assignation for Thursday with an adorable hooker. The rest of Wednesday passed the same as Monday and Tuesday had done, in the haze of paraphilic fugue state.

Thursday morning, genital arousal and paraphilic imagery prevailed. My masochized brain craved the stimulation my new dominatrix would provide. When Sarah arrived, she was willing to play the part of a dominatrix, although she wasn't a sadist. Of course, Sarah's role is secondary, but my casting of her is primary. After all, I'm the one who is in need of an orgasm, not her.

Sarah's role was to tease and tantalize me, but not allow any touching between us. Her flared thighs were a perfect match to my lovemap. Inches before my eyes, Sarah exhibited her labial cleft. I yearned to lick her hole of lust. My erect penis panted. Yet I was not allowed to touch my penis. The stimulation seemed intolerable. My genital fluid poured onto the floor.

Since there is, for me, an interconnection between genital arousal and punishment, Sarah found an arbitrary cause to spank me. She directed me to lie across a pillow, with my extremity of lust tucked between my thighs. Then Sarah bound both my wrists and ankles. Combined with words of admonishment, she strapped my bare rump with a belt. The impact of the leather against my tender skin was fantastically agonizing. As reenacted from childhood, and from recurrent imagery, the whipping is ideal. Then, the restaged scenario transforms excruciating pain into psychophysical ecstasy. This stage of masochism is more ideal than heaven.

When my reddened buttocks had received one hundred lashes, my temporary dominatrix untied my hands and feet. I had ejaculated twice. Later, we enjoyed dinner together. Sarah wanted to replace my Baltimore mistress, Dawn. I promised to phone Sarah whenever I'd return to Pittsburgh. Although Sarah didn't realize it, I would be achieving orgasms over her physique and demeanor for at least another week. She aroused me in absentia, without fee.

Friday morning, my welted buttocks facilitated more orgasms. Afterward, I managed to watch television and eat my second meal of the week. Finally, I sensed my body and mind beginning to normalize. I phoned my mistress in Baltimore. We bandied words of lust. Dawn's voice over the phone induced more penile swelling. That night, my masochized imagery shunted between the salacious images of both Sarah and Dawn. My genital fluid did not decrease. My orgasms were still ejaculatory.

Saturday morning, I repacked my property and tried to salvage my sales week. Amazingly, I performed quite well that day. In short, my sales in one day equaled what I might have accomplised in an ordinary week. I counted my earnings, and departed for Baltimore. Dawn would be expecting me, and that's all I cared about. I was living from the last orgasm to the next orgasm, on and on.

What I'm about to disclose offers, perhaps, a tenable explanation as to how inanimate things can seem animate. It occurred about twenty-five years ago. I was alone while walking through a wooded area. I felt the presage of a masochized orgasm. This arcane feeling was experienced as a tingling in my flaccid penis. Mysteriously, the sticks on the ground and on the trees beckoned me. Pervading my mental screen were images of protruding buttocks. The sticks seemed to urge me to thrash myself. I kept walking in an effort to ignore the sadomasochistic lust.

Subsequently, the ideation of whipping myself dominated my mental stage. The distorted ideation and imagery of my mind disposed me to whipping myself, thereby performing the scenes represented on my mind's stage. Suddenly, my walking was impaired. Rapidly my penis engorged with blood. A circuit of sensation flowed between my masochistic imagery and my genitals. I grasped a stick with which to whip myself, but I had not given my informed consent. I wanted to scream for help, but how would I explain it? Moreover, it would be too embarrassing to admit what was happening.

As a result of this insistent lust, I lowered my pants next to a tree in the forest. I worried about being discovered, but I couldn't resist. With a sturdy stick in my right hand, I lashed my naked buttocks. After beating my buttocks slowly, I increased the stinging strokes. Soon, my bare buttocks were covered with welts.

The paraphilic stimulus was, once again, overwhelming. My arm ached from pounding my own buttocks. My penile fluid drooled onto the leaves under the trees. Oddly, I was disturbed with myself, for I couldn't beat my buttocks harshly enough. Permeating my mind and body was the transformation from pain to ecstasy. In fact, no drug on earth could equal or exceed my masochistic euphoria.

When my masochized ejaculation occurred, I dropped the stick and collapsed in orgasmic exhaustion. Gazing through the tops of the trees, I said to myself: "Where is my free will?" My monologue continued with: "I'm supposed to be the master of my fate and the captain of my soul; what's wrong? I'm feeling so good, but this is so wrong."

Later that night, and throughout the week, my red buttocks facilitated many orgasms. The mere reflection of my red rump was enough to trigger genital arousal when viewed in the mirror. After this paraphilic episode, my extremity of lust remained semi-erect for several days. In that state, I was isolated. I kept my secret to myself. If I talked, who would understand?

The scenario of this paraphilic fugue resurfaced throughout the next ten years of my life. Contemplating its power, I supposed that someone might attribute it to spirits in the trees. Those spirits of lust invaded me.

The paraphilic fugue will strike anytime and anywhere, and totally without warning. As a train shunts from one track to another, so do I shunt from my everyday situation to the paraphilic fugue. For example, there was a large weeping willow tree in someone's yard. As I drove by that yard and observed the flowing branches of the weeping willow, I experienced a sudden urge to stop my car. In my mind were dramatic scenes of being whipped with a cane from a similar tree. My genitals swelled instantly, but the paraphilic fugue didn't take over, that time. Perhaps the whole tree gave only an attenuated beckoning, as compared with a cane for whipping.

There was one occasion when a paraphilic fugue struck in a hardware store. The cleaning product I marketed sold in hardware stores from coast to coast, and I rarely missed any of the ones in between. Wearing my three-piece suit, I entered a store that sold both hardware and marine supplies. The owner was busy. Then my eyes glanced at an upright box containing thin pieces of wood. Suddenly, my penis began swelling, and my mind inflated with imagery of being spanked by the pieces of wood. In less than one minute, the ooze from my penis marked the trouser leg of my suit. Instead of selling my product, I departed to my car quickly. Fortunately, the effect of this paraphilic fugue diminished shortly thereafter.

Another episode of the paraphilic fugue was a case of lust at first sight. It was early in the day, within the town of Freehold, New Jersey. Earnestly, my intention was to break my previous sales records. This town presented many good prospects for optimal sales. Usually, when I aim to achieve an ideal day of sales, I accomplish it. I try to ignore those fortuitous events over which I have no control.

I stepped into a newsstand. I find markets for my polishing cloths everywhere. The owner purchased my product for personal use, not to market. Subsequently I scanned the magazines. Some of them were magazines of erotica. Naturally, I was inclined to view the erotic pictorials. I glanced at them, but I didn't want to be distracted, so I returned the magazine to the rack.

Selling commenced quite well, but then I experienced mental images of a specific girl posed in the magazine's pictorial. My attempt to ignore its arousing effect was futile. Intrusive images of her flashed across my mental screen. However, whereas the girl's pictorial showed pubic hair, my mind's image of her showed a hairless pudenda. Accordingly, my penis swelled.

Unable to conceal the manifestation of lust, I walked back to my car. I couldn't sell. I was angry and confused. I yearned for a new car, a house, and money in the bank. My paraphilia, demanding its own expression, defeated me.

Seated within my car in a crowded parking lot, I wished that I could defeat my paraphilia. Perhaps death would deprive it of another victory, but even suicide eluded me. Ambivalently, I realized that achieving orgasm was the only way to cope. Moreover, a masturbatory orgasm was the only maneuver that lay under my control. After all, an orgasm would allow me to continue selling, and that's what I desired.

Starting my car, I drove out of the crowded parking lot. I needed to locate a private place to appease my paraphilia. While driving, my intuition posed a few interesting thoughts: if I were a pedophilic rapist, I'd be seeing a prepubertal girl to rape. If I were a lust murderer, I'd be seeking a pubertal or older woman to rape and kill. However, my orgasm didn't need a victim. I was glad of that.

A church parking lot was vacant. When I reflected upon that church, I recalled my divorce. Furthermore, I yearned to share my sexual feelings with a lover. However, this present genital arousal actually impeded my love affairs. Lying with a woman who cared for me and nurtured me is what I needed. I longed to love and be loved, but this pending orgasm was beyond love.

After achieving an ejaculatory orgasm, I felt euphoric. Yet, I'd lost several hours of selling with its potential profit. "If only I had someone to turn to," I thought, "might I be helped?"

Nora was a good, but incomplete, match to my lovemap. Many years I'd spent in coital activity with her. However, paraphilic fugues care nothing about wholesome, two-partnered lust. The paraphilic fugue seeks its own methods of unwholesome lust.

One night Nora needed a place to sleep with her son. I let them lodge at my apartment. The opportunity to copulate with her that night would have been easy. She was genitally aroused as frequently as I was. However, I experienced an eerie inquietude. I sensed the onset of a paraphilic fugue. Although I wanted to stay there, with Nora and her son, I couldn't. I posed the excuse that I needed to be alone for awhile.

As I drove toward a Holiday Inn, I felt irascible and tense. Invading my mental screen were arousing forms. At first, the lusty images were desultory. Then, only images of buttocks. My genital arousal overwhelmed me. Registering at the hotel was difficult, for my hand trembled. When I entered my room, collapsing on the bed was all I could do. I tossed my head on the pillow, as the paraphilic invader altered my consciousness.

Cast onto my mental screen were masochistic images, pear-shaped buttocks positioned for spanking. They beckoned me to participate in being spanksed. My penis was engorged. My paraphilic brain insisted that I whip my own buttocks. A self-imposed whipping will facilitate the burst of orgasm.

Removing my belt from my trousers, I knelt in front of an armchair. My left arm and head was pressed against the cushion. With my right arm, I held the belt. Then I commenced lashing my naked buttocks. At first, my body flinched from the sting of the leather belt. Thrashing my buttocks continued until the skin was turned red and sore. The swinging strap, with accompanying images, kept on until there was no pain.

The transformation from pain to ecstasy was warm and truly wonderful. With all my strength, I had lashed my burning buttocks, and I now felt euphoric. I despised having to achieve an orgasm this way, but it surely felt good—so good, so exhausting, and so immobilizing, I couldn't move. And my penis literally couldn't deflate.

More images entered my mental stage. Imagery of girls without panties, and especially girls without pubic hair, rearoused my penis. I gazed at their vulvar clefts, and oozed onto the carpet. Within that state, I achieved another orgasm. I felt "high."

The sensitized skin of my buttocks, and the masochistic imagery of my mind induced repeated orgasms until it was time to check out the next day. I returned to my apartment. Nora complained about my absence. What could I tell her? I couldn't explain my absence even to myself.

One night, I drifted through the bars of Baltimore's Block and entered the Pussy Cat Club. Dancing on stage was a shapely girl with brown hair. Suddenly, I couldn't leave that club.

When the stripteaser finished her dance, she disappeared for a while, then reemerged with her coat, as though departing. As she walked by my stool, I invited her to sit with me. Her name was Dawn, and her face, demeanor, and physique were parallel to some dominatrix images of my mind, although I didn't know it at that moment of our first encounter. I explained what I needed and proposed a price. Dawn was surprised, for most men procure her for coital activity, not posing in private.

Later she met me at the Holiday Inn on Rt. 40. Dawn had inhabited my imagery since the moment I observed her at the club. Naturally, my genitalia swelled and remained swollen. Although she reported her age to be eighteen, she didn't look any more than sixteen. Nonetheless, it was a precocious sixteen. Her posing for me was tendered at seventy-five dollars.

Dawn exhibited her vulvar cleft, buttocks, and breasts for me in tantalizing poses. My brain had discovered its stimulus, but without respect for me.

That night, I spent about eight hours in masturbatory fantasy. Mentally, I was stimulated by her form and figure. Then the images of her confected another scenario. Dawn became my imaginal dominatrix. I imagined her ordering me across her lap. She was forceful as she spanked me. Penile fluid flowed as I vividly imaged her spanking me, fiercely. Although I didn't understand it completely, something connected the scenario of my mind with my impaired and distorted relationship in pairbonding with my mother. Subsequently, my penis ejaculated with orgasmic ecstasy. It seemed strange to feel so good.

As a result, the next time I spoke with Dawn, I asked her to play the role of my dominatrix. She agreed at the cost of a hundred dollars per session. In order to maintain complete control over me, Dawn allowed me to ejaculate in her vagina, but only when she permitted it. Moreover, ejaculation had to be at the moment of her demanding it. Penile penetration could be only as deep or as prolonged as she decided.

Since the paraphilic fugue is an altered state of mind, and I never stopped experiencing that state with Dawn for two years, one might say that I lived in the paraphilic fugue. Except for the masochistic ritual and distorted attachment of my own paraphilic fugue, being in love is the same.

Dawn danced erotically at several clubs. One night, after a day of sales, I visited her at the Flamingo Club. My genital arousal had been active throughout that day. Contrary to Dawn's direct orders, I fondled my genitalia. She forbade the touching on my penis even in the shower. Dawn promised to whip me with a strap if I fondled my penis. Her restriction actually incited genital touching.

When interrogated about fingering my penis during that day, I confessed, but complained about not being allowed to touch it. Well, Dawn didn't like being disobeyed. She ordered me to the rear of the club. Behind curtains, she removed my belt from my trousers. I knelt on a cushioned bench, and projected my buttocks. When the music of the club played loudly, Dawn commenced beating my bare buttocks. Since Dawn was particularly angry, she whipped me accordingly. Several minutes of lashing prevailed before she paused. Then, when the music continued, she continued strapping me. Frequently, the end of the strap would strike my scrotum. I flinched, but she ignored my pain.

Up until my masochistic metamorphosis overcame me, I was slightly apprehensive about someone discovering our masochistic ritual. But once my masochistic euphoria did occur, nothing else on earth mattered.

In order to keep Dawn near me, I hired her to drive my car. I traveled about three thousand miles per week. She made a perfect chauffeur. Furthermore, she performed as the perfect dominatrix for me. I lived under Dawn's rule and relished it. That is, my masochized self relished it. Otherwise, I never would have behaved as I did with her.

My sales were prolific in West Virginia. My erotic brain yearned for orgasmic fulfillment. Dawn was determined to control me. She knew that I'd had a hard-on since I'd awakened that morning. So, she gave me a quota to reach in sales. If I didn't reach her monetary quota, she'd restrict my orgasm. Additionally, my hands were to avoid any contact with my semierect penis.

Not touching my genitals was impossible. Then Dawn stopped the car on the shoulder of the highway. Yes, even while parked on the side of the road, she disciplined me. Dawn ordered my pants down. She folded my leather belt. Then, ordering me to sit on my hands, she lashed my swollen penis. Amazingly, nothing stopped her from beating my penis, not even me. Can you imagine someone lashing your erect penis or your vulva? Without the altered state of the paraphilic fugue, I couldn't have endured the pain.

Although my punishnent was severe, Dawn made me bend over the car seat. Then, with cars passing by, she lashed my buttocks. While she strapped my buttocks, my penile fluid flowed like a stream. My masochistic euphoria made the embarrassing situation worth every second.

Irrespective of my activities, a spontaneous image of Dawn on my mental screen would engorge my penis. At times, my mental theater would stage a scenario. Then it would spur me to enact that scenario with the actual Dawn. One such scene took place at Duke's Motel, just outside of Baltimore City.

Inhabiting my paraphilic imagery were scenes of Dawn beating my erect penis. Dawn was expected to spank me that day. Spanking me frequently was her way of both satisfying her sadism, and earning about six hundred dollars per week. Likewise, my masochism was satisfied.

When Dawn arrived, I conveyed subliminal messages to her. I felt disposed to having my penis beaten. Although I didn't want my erect penis lashed with a belt, the urge was irrepressible. I watched her undress. Dawn teased me, the swelling of my genitals felt wonderful. Then, she allowed me to slide my penile erection into her vagina. I thrust it only as deep as she'd allow. This time, she made me stop when I sensed an imminent orgasm. She told me to stand at the side of the bed.

Furthermore, with a sadistic look on her face, Dawn began beating my engorged penis. Although it was difficult to stand in position while she lashed my penis, I knew what it would lead to. She whipped every part of my body in proximity of my groin. Then, out of determination to force compliance to her will, she switched to the other end of the belt; the end with the buckle.

Dawn required my stationary obedience as she lashed my genitalia with the belt buckle. I recalled being whipped with a belt buckle in my childhood. Then, the belt buckle struck my testicles. The sudden surge of pain caused my body to collapse. That elicited Dawn's compassion. She inquired about taking me to the hospital. Strangely, I felt comforted by the very person who had inflicted the intense pain in my testicles. Soon that pain was also transformed into euphoria. It was amazing, and far beyond any previous masochistical event I had experienced. Although I couldn't utter the words, I did not want her to cease thrashing me. The pleasure/pain principle has ambiguous validity.

Subsequently, Dawn's partnership with me waned. As in any partnership, there must be a reciprocal attachment, even when it is distorted. Dawn's tolerance for inflicting pain was exhausted. Our vandalized lovemaps no longer reciprocated each other.

Illogically, but paraphilically, I strived to retain Dawn's role as dominatrix. I felt just like the battered wife returning to the abusive husband for more abuse. In fact, it's the same.

Dawn turned eighteen at the end of our relationship. Her disposition was a match to my mother's disposition, especially when she was angry. At eighteen, Dawn's face matched my image of my mother's face.

In 1964, I enrolled in a seminary. At the time, I believed this event in my life to be a design of the God of Christendom. I was a dedicated Christian. I memorized the Scriptures. There was no deficiency in my Christian ethics or belief. Nonetheless, something was wrong.

If there are Christians reading this manifestation of my paraphilia, they'll be inclined to swear that the devil caused it. If the Apostle Paul could read this, he'd conclude that it is the sin that dwells within me. I who have experienced it know it to be the outcome of vandalism of my lovemap, manifested characteristically as masochism.

The seminary was an old stone church. The rooms were about the same size as my prison cell. Each was heated by an old iron radiator. That radiator was an inanimate object. Or was it? Each day when I returned from class, it seemed to beckon me. It beckoned without uttering a word, move, or change of form. I found myself seeking to know the source of the power that the radiator had over me, for power it certainly possessed.

Nightly, I studied theology. Nightly, my penis erected. I had no erotica to view or read. Still my penis swelled and oozed to an imagined scenario of naked buttocks. Frequently, I broke the vow of abstinence and masturbated to diminish the erotic tension, so as to return to my studies. Each fix was only temporary.

While lying in bed one night, I had an eidetic image of a scene in which my buttocks were pressing against the radiator. Instantly, my penis swelled. How great would be an orgasm achieved by the heat from the radiator? To suppress such sinful speculation, I prayed, and I prayed. "Please help me," I prayed. I automatically assumed that the devil had something to do with such distorted feeling. I knew that my faith was strong enough to fight the demon in the radiator. I knew that God would save me, for his word conveyed that promise.

Ignorant of sexology, I assumed that copulating with a hooker would dispel my phallic lust. Perhaps that was God's message to me, I reflected. So I sought and located a hooker. The images of my mental screen as we copulated were the same as when I masturbated. It was not the hooker's physique that spurred my lust to its goal of orgasm. It was my private imagery.

My masochism had deceived me. My paraphilic ideation and imagery came together in a scenario of satisfying the urge to burn my buttocks on the radiator. Then, perhaps, I wouldn't be so frustrated. I knew that I couldn't resist. I wondered how thrilling the orgasm might be.

Late one night, the radiator disturbed my sleep. My room was extremely hot and the air was dry. There was a clanging in the water pipes. My mind was rehearsing a scenario of how to proceed with a hot spot orgasm, courtesy of the radiator.

The room was densely dark. I supposed that it was occupied by a demon. I tugged my shorts off. Kneeling with my buttocks a few inches from the hot radiator, I paused. I knew from my early childhood that the pain would transform into ecstasy, but that its onset would provoke reluctance. "Could my God be in the same room with this demon?" I questioned.

Pressing my naked buttocks against the radiator, I proceeded cautiously. My rigid penis seemed as hard as the coils of the radiator. Fluid oozed onto the wooden floors "Why do I do this stupid thing?" I asked myself. The answer was a transformation that took place in stages. By the time the initial pain had passed, my mind and body were ecstatic. I didn't want to stop. Finally, my ejaculation gushed onto the floor, I was in highest heaven. The demon felt wonderful.

Thereafter, I returned to my masochistic orgasm nightly. Guilty feelings overcame me. Praying didn't help. I needed to talk to someone. So I explained my frequent masturbation to my theology teacher. I realized that I couldn't remain in the seminary. With a great magnitude of despair, I abandoned my belief in the concept of God. If there were a God, surely God would have saved me. But there was no salvation, neither from the demon nor the radiator. God did not even know about the paraphilic fugue state, and that the religious principle of punishment had predisposed me to the paraphilia of masochism.

If I do things by voluntary choice, then why do I do them? If I don't do things by choice, then why do they happen? The explanation for the occurrence of the radiator ritual can only be that I was transported into an altered state of consciousness, a paraphilic fugue.

My Christianized life had begun while I was in the army, somewhere in Germany, during 1963. Like everyone else, I was seeking an answer to the question of the meaning to life. I thought that I had discovered it in Christianity. I had excellent help. A missionary from the Navigators dedicated much of his time to my growth as a Christian. His emphasis was upon memorization of the Holy Bible. I memorized at least ten verses per week, and I practiced memorizing verses for over a year. Needless to say, I knew my God through Holy Scriptures.

In the army I was the company mail clerk and keeper of protective masks. The protective masks were stored in the basement of Taylor Barracks, located on the base on which I lived. That storage room was ideal for studying the Bible. I had enrolled in a Bible study course from Moody Bible Institute. I studied daily. I performed quite well. I had had an active mind.

Spontaneous mental images and ideas outside of Bible study worked in my brain recurrently. They were of females buttocks, and they swelled my penis. Replays of eroticized scenes became persistent, followed by arousal. Desperate in the hope that masturbation would dislodge my intrusive imagery, I indulged in it aplenty, and at the same time swore to resist it.

Eventually, my imaginal scenarios became quite disturbing. I experienced embarrassing ideas and images of inserting a small flashlight into my anal canal. I resisted them as absurd. Finally, the imagery and ideation of self-imposed anal penetration overpowered my resistance. "How can something I don't want possess me so ardently?" I wondered. Then my vandalized lovemap confected a scenario of how to proceed with this distorted lust.

Hesitantly, I turned off the lights. My body trembled and my genitals swelled intensely. I lowered my fatigue pants, and reclined on the concrete floors. This anal urging vexed me greatly, but resisting didn't work. While inserting the small flashlight into my anal canal, I wondered what I was supposed to feel. When the flashlight became entrenched within my rectum, penile fluid flowed onto the floor. Imagery of penetrating a vagina filled my mental stage. With my eyes closed, I imagined myself copulating the anal canal of a female. My own experience of being penetrated was imaged as penetrating her.

The climax was ecstatic. The muscles of my anus ejected the flashlight. I worried about the implications. Since anal copulation is a practice of intermale lust, I feared that I'd become homosexual.

Temporarily, my urging for self-imposed anal penetration substituted for my masochistic urge for self-imposed spankings. I stopped worrying about becoming homosexual, for I didn't have any male images inciting me to penile lust. My paraphilic imagery and ideation always paralleled my paraphilic rituals and enactments with a female.

Next, my paraphilia of masochism confected a scenario with anal penetration. Meanwhile, I prayed to God through Jesus Christ. Optimistically, I prayed that my newest imagery wouldn't actualize itself. I thought that I was closer to God, for I had recently spoken in tongues. Perhaps God was testing me, I conjectured.

One day while studying the Scriptures, penile arousal again distracted me. I had a vision of my buttocks being lashed while my anus held the small flashlight. I proceeded to enact that masochistic ritual as though I had no other choice.

Lying on the floor, I inserted the flashlight into my snug anus. With my right arm, I commenced thrashing my bared buttocks. At first, I strapped my behind with a belt, but it didn't sting enough for a maximum orgasm. So, I whipped my rump with an extension cord, which burned intensely. Mentally, I was penetrating a girl's rectum while being whipped. Spreading the cheeks of my buttocks, I whipped the sensitive skin between my cheeks. The masochistic euphoria of that exercise was unparalleled. My orgasm was a tornado touching down.

Paraphilia Imagined

The paraphilic images of my mind have dictated my behavior. However, there had to have been a niche in my mind for the actual image to fit into. The following imaginal scenario was the outcome of viewing a magazine pictorial while in prison. My eyes glanced at it, then I examined it closely, a pictorial of an auburn-haired girl. Afterward, my mind's view observed her on my inner stage. I spontaneously experienced penile arousal. The image of the auburn-haired girl was arousing me from within my own mind. But I didn't put her likeness in my mind's view. What do I want with girls on my mental stage when I can't touch them? What can I do with penile arousal in a prison cell?

More importantly, why didn't one of the other girls from the magazine pictorial lodge herself on my mental stage? If I had a choice, I'd imagine Loni Anderson. I've tried to be orgasmic over her, but I can't be. There isn't any niche in my lovemap for her. Being in love or falling in love is without my choice, will, or preference. And that is irrespective of whether or not my lovemap has been vandalized, as in fact it has.

This is rehearsal. The story that you're about to read is my sexual brain rehearsing me for a possible role. The same type of rehearsal preceded my lust affair with Connie. Specifically, a vandalized lovemap rehearsed me for unconditional obedience to her. That rehearsal was then actually staged or materialized when I escorted Connie into the orgasmic armed robberies.

I was housed on the fourth floor of the prison. I reclined on my bunk with the light out. When my eyes closed, a mental image of the auburn-haired girl appeared. She is seated on a bar stool. My imaginal self approaches her at the bar. She says her name is Sandy. Lustiness pervades me. When I seat myself next to her, she looks directly at my erect penis, which protrudes from within my trousers. "Did I do that?" inquires Sandy, as she touches the material that restrains it. "Yes, that's what your tantalizing form does to me," I say and I tremble in her alluring presence.

Fictively, my ears long to hear dominating words. My skin yearns to feel the stinging and burning from a paddle or strap. My eyes crave the view of her naked crotch. My knees want to kneel in front of her worshipfully. I'll give her anything to be my auburn-haired dominatrix.

Sandy has an aura of confidence, which permeates me. "What kind of girl do you like?" she adds as though she already knows about my tendency toward a dominant mistress. "Well, I don't know if I like it, but I need a dominatrix," I reply. At the same moment, fluid pours from my engorged penis. "I don't know if you'll be a good slave. I require total obedience," Sandy says, as she stares into my face waiting for a reply.

In a state of overstimulation, I disclose my former lust affairs. I reveal my own terms of capitulating to her as my dominatrix.

"I'd rather lie across your lap and be spanked than do anything else," I explain. Eventually, we walk out of the bar and get into my Rolls-Royce. By that time, my trouser leg is sticky from penile fluid. Sandy feels the wetness of my trouser material, and says, "This will merit your first spanking. When we arrive at your house, you will take your pants off so they can dry. Then come to me." Her forecast of a spanking induces my penis to secrete more fluid.

After arriving at my imaginal home, we look at some of its rooms. My entire body is filled with lustful tension. Removing my pants to let them dry, I wipe the gooey fluid from my genitalia. Proceeding toward the room where Sandy is waiting, I wonder how harshly she spanks a man. Once I have entered the room, I gaze at my new mistress. I long to know how much a good spanking will burn and sting my buttocks.

Sandy raises her skirt to expose her naked crotch. My erect penis is extremely rigid. "Get down on your knees," she orders, as she spreads her thighs widely in front of my face. Obeying her is the easiest thing I've ever done. She looks like the goddess of all womankind. Overarousal pervades me.

"Get across my lap," Sandy says, pointing to her lap. I drape myself across her naked thighs, and position my erect penis between her legs. She orders me to stay in position. The strap with which she lashes my buttocks burns intensely. After approximately one hundred lashes, she ceases her punishment.

I am euphoric, ecstatic, and orgasmic. Sandy's beating on my buttocks has sent me into a transported state of masochism. Now she orders me onto my knees directly in front of her cavern of lust. "This is the kind of mistress I'll be," she said, as she teases me with her cuntal lips. I want nothing else of life, except to be enslaved by her. I had achieved one orgasm while she spanked me, but my penis is still erect. "You may jerk off if you like, but don't get any of that stuff on me," she says, as she moves her succulent cunt closer to the edge of the chair. Twenty minutes of masturbation later, another ejaculation occurs. "Now go get a towel and wipe your sperm off the floor," Sandy orders, taking charge.

There I was, on my bunk in a cell, and I had just had the most wonderful orgasm. Before this imaginal scenario of Sandy faded in the weeks ahead, I viewed at least sixty more episodes. I was hyperorgasmic, and all within the confines of a prison cell. I did what most inmates do with their time. If they're rapists, they mentally rehearse raping girls, or in some cases males. If they're sadists, they rehearse beating their girlfriends, wives, and whores. The state pays for it! When they're released, they simply perform what they have rehearsed. If they're paraphilic murderers, their mental scenarios rehearse them for murder, but their years of mental rehearsal will improve their methods of killing and avoidance of detection. There is no special motivation to rehearsal imagery. It simply happens.

I call my rehearsals mental videotapes. The one you have just read is available for my future viewing. In future viewings it will carry the same theme, but with scenarios that vary inexhaustibly. There's no reality so vivid and powerful as having your imagination run wild. A mental scenario of masochism will always be a scenario of masochism. I've transposed into words my mental videotape of sadomasochism. Now, I'll disclose another mental videotape. But I'm not the actor in this one.

I've reclined on my bunk. In my mind's view, I see a farm with a large barn, a chicken house, and a silo. In the farmhouse kitchen, I see a teenage girl. She has long, blonde hair, a pear-shaped rump, a slender waist, a sloped nose, shapely legs and thighs, and full, cone-shaped breasts. She's wearing a skimpy dress. "Donna, are you finished washing those dishes?" her mother asks, as she enters the kitchen. Before Donna can reply, her mother slaps her across the buttocks. Donna jumps from the sting inflicted by her mother. "Mom, I'll be done in just a minute," she says, as a tear rolls down her cheek.

"You're too damn slow, I'll have to whip your ass," her mother threatens, and she goes to fetch a strap to whip Donna's buttocks. Donna has finished the dishes by the time her mother returns with the strap, but it makes no difference. Seeing the wide leather strap evokes terror in Donna. "No, mommy, please don't whip me again," she says, and backs into a corner.

The cruel mother orders Donna's panties off, and tells her to lie across a kitchen chair. Tugging her panties off, Donna drapes herself across the chair. My mind's view of her buttocks induces a discharge of fluid from my rigid erection. I watch as the mother commences strapping her daughter's skin. Soon Donna's rump is bright red and welted from the swinging leather strap. "Lie still or I'll whip your ass all day," says her mother. Donna's hands grasp the legs of the chair. She strives to be still during her mother's beating. When the mother's arm reaches exhaustion, the strapping ceases.

Afterward, Donna goes to her room. She examines her beaten butt in a mirror. It is so sore that it hurts her to sit on her bed. Meanwhile, she cries herself to sleep. In the next scene, her older brother enters her bedroom. Donna's panties are still on the kitchen floor. Quickly she sits up on her bed while attempting to conceal her naked crotch.

"You know, mom will whip your ass if I report that you're not wearing panties," says her brother, as he moves closer to where she sits on the bed. Donna pleads with him not to report her. "What's in it for me if I don't say anything?" he asks. He longs to peek between her naked thighs. Donna turns her back to him and exposes the result of mother's whipping. Her brother really doesn't care about her sore tail.

Whimpering, Donna bargains with him. "Bobbie, please don't say that you saw me without panties. I'll let you look between my thighs if you promise not to say anything," she says. She raises her skimpy slip above her slender waist. He stares in amazement, looking at Donna's salacious vulva. "Is this better?" she asks, as she leans back and spreads her luring limbs widely. Bobbie drops to his knees beside her bed. He gazes at her pink hole. While being tantalized by Donna's delicious cunt, he masturbates. It is the best orgasm he has ever experienced.

In the next scene, it's late at night. Donna is sleeping. Her bedroom door opens. Her father steps into her room and closes the door behind him. Seating himself on the edge of her bed, he rubs her rump from atop the blanket. Donna wakes up and is surprised to see her father seated on the bed, especially to feel his hand on her butt. "Now just be quiet," her father cautions, as he pulls the blanket from her body. Donna still isn't wearing panties. "Bobbie told me that you have a real pretty pussy. How about showing it to me?" her father cajoles, with an eager look on his face.

Donna turns onto her back. Parting her legs widely, she prsents her titilating vulva to his view. Her father, equipped with a small flashlight, directs the beam of light directly at her crotch. He is overwhelmed with lust. "If you do me a favor, I'll prevent your mother from whipping you as much as she does," he says. Her eyes widen with curiosity. She yearns to know what kind of favor would diminish the frequency of being whipped. "Have you ever sucked a man's penis?" he said, unzipping his jeans. "Daddy, I don't know how to mouth a penis," she protests gazing in surprise at the length of her father's cock. "You wanna keep from being whipped, don't you?" her father replies, as he presents his erection to his daughter's mouth. Reluctantly, she licks the head of his lusty organ. He encourages her to slide her open mouth over the head of it. Cautiously, she lets it enter her mouth. When she feels it bump the back of her throat, she commences mouthing it slowly. Her father's body shudders from the contact of her gentle mouth on his phallus.

Donna's mind is frenzied. She has never engulfed the length of a man's penis before. Her father is anxious for an orgasm. Placing a hand on her head, he commences thrusting his extremity of lust to the rear of her mouth. Submissively, she permits his powerful penis to slide in and out of her mouth. Fifteen minutes of oral copulation later, her father shudders as he ejaculates into her warm mouth.

With several gulps, Donna swallows his sticky come. He is exhausted. "Daddy, you'll keep your promise, won't you?" beseeches Donna, holding her slip at her waist. He agrees to prevent any more whippings for another week. Of course, he vows to return.

In the next scene, a week has gone by. There is a delivery man who barters certain farm products with Donna's mother. Budget money is limited. Calling Donna into the kitchen, her mother instructs her on how to behave toward the delivery man. To elicit full cooperation, her mother promises to suspend Donna's punishments if she is cooperative. "Al wants to peek under your skirt," her mother explains. "I'll invite him into the living room. Afterward, you go in there, too, and I'll leave you two alone. Be nice to him." Her mother glances through the kitchen window to see if the delivery man has arrived.

"I guess it's better to be sacrificed than whipped," Donna muses, as she examines her clothing to see if she looks good for Al. Outside, there is the sound of a truck arriving. Mother is on the porch. She greets Al. Donna watches from the window while her mother speaks with Al. "I wonder if he will do more than look at me," Donna thinks, reflecting on her experiences with her brother and father.

Mother and Al enter the kitchen. Mother carries several packages; the result of having bartered with Al. "Oh, well, it's time for me," Donna supposes, as she prances into the living room where mother and Al are waiting. Donna seats herself directly across from Al's view. This time there is no concern about exposing her panties. As previously planned, her mother leaves Donna alone with Al.

"You want to look at my panties?" asks Donna, as she rises and stands directly in front of Al's chair. She smiles as she raises the hem of her skirt. Holding her skirt above the waist, she watches Al's genital excitement. "I had no idea that men got so excited from looking at a girl's panties," Donna teases, as she watches Al rub his jeans where his penis presses against the material. Suddenly, Al's body quakes in orgasm. "Mother can't be angry with me now that he's had a good orgasm," Donna tells herself in an interior monologue. She drops the hem of her skirt.

The preceding episode ended when I myself achieved an orgasm in my jailhouse cell. There are hundreds of episodes to this type of my mental videotape. I've labeled this scoptophilic sadomasochism, for I'm viewing scenes showing sexual and sadomasochostic behavior by other people. The fact that I'm not a performer is significant—I am watching.

In another mental videotape, I am an actor, performer, and spectator. The scenario begins as I walk on the street of Baltimore's Block. I had experienced an urge to view a naked and specific type of body. It was an irresistible sensation. I walk from bar to bar searching for the ideal lady with the right body. Eventually I enter the right bar. There she stands in a black leotard. The conformation of her bodily parts matches specific images in my mind.

While she dances, I ask the bartender who she is. Cindy is her name. When her music stops, she sits with another customer. A few minutes later, she accompanies the customer to the rear of the bar. Approximately ten minutes later, they return to the bar. My lust for viewing her is driving me crazy. She sits on a bar stool only a few places from me. I stare in her direction to get her attention. It works. She leaves her stool and seats herself next to me.

I purchase two drinks. I use a hundred-dollar bill to buy them. When I receive the change, I push it across the bar's counter in her direction. Being a smart girl, she guesses what the money implies. I explain my fixation for viewing the vulvas of adolescent girls. "That's all you want, is to look at my pussy?" Cindy asks, with a perplexed look on her pretty face. We move to the rear of the bar.

Locating a corner with privacy, she unsnaps the crotch of her leotard. Facing me, she parts her shapely thighs. The view of her gorgeous groin stimulates my sexual brain. Parting the lips of her labia, she exposes more of her vulva. Somehow viewing is intensely more stimulating to me than coital activity. Before departing, I tip her with a hundred-dollar bill. To me, viewing her alluring body has been sublimely better than achieving an orgasm.

Episodes like this have been recurrent for twenty years on my mental stage. Watching the mental videotape ends when I achieve an orgasm. I achieve an orgasm without viewing any images of heterosexual copulation or interpersonal contact. In fact, to be orgasmic a fantasy doesn't need to include genital activity of any type, except that one of the sexes, myself, is experiencing a fantasy.

I'm a paraphile. I have theorized a method to alter my paraphilic criminal behavior. Up until 1990, my mind played the preceding scenarios to induce orgasm. Subsequently, from the outset of 1990, my sexual brain produced three different mental scenarios. They are depictions of pairing, partnering, and love's pairbonding. My orgasmic frequency diminished to once per week from ten per week. Now my imagination is deluged with scenes of pairbonded affectionate love, whereas before my mind's imagery staged only scenes of paraphilic lust.

5

Born into Hell
Imprinting for a Paraphilic Lifetime

My mother was educated in an inadequate country school. She came from a family of nine children on an old farm. She was a pretty lady.

Reportedly, her father was abusive to his children, and justified his child abuse as punishment. Naturally, this idea of atonement through pain and punishment was carried on by my parent. Of course, parental terrorism was endorsed by the Book of Proverbs in the Christian Bible.

My mother was about twenty-one at my birth. I had two older sisters and one older brother. The siblings were born like this: sister, brother, sister, and myself. Many years later, there was another brother. My mother didn't need a fourth child, and my sisters didn't want another brother. Of course, no one considered that I didn't ask to be born. Consequently, my sisters and mother condemned me for being, whereas I didn't ask to be.

My nescient mother didn't teach me about this predatory world. How could she? She didn't know any better herself. I grew up in her distorted world. She knew little about human sexuality, and even less about little boys.

Though she was a manic-depressive, she didn't know it. Genetically, she passed it on to me. Unfortunately, I didn't know of my manic-depressive condition until it was too late. Yet, I'm now held accountable.

I was born toward the end of the Second World War. My father was in combat during that war. He came from an idealistic family.

According to his mother, I didn't have the proper morphology to be from her side of the family, irrespective of my birthright.

My father claims to be stoical, which manifests itself as refined macho manhood. Ideally, a male must live up to his criterion of manhood or he is not a man, irrespective of his genitals. That's tough on a little boy.

After four episodes of gestation and lactation, my mother's feminine figure was altered. So, when my father returned from combat, he didn't experience the same erotic/genital arousal for my mother as he had done before. Consequently, his ephebophilic lovemap hooked him up with another woman, much younger, leaving four helpless children behind.

Apparently my father's second wife was a mismatch, especially since he subsequently married her daughter. Prior to that lascivious episode, he returned to impregnate my mother with a fifth unwanted child. His coital insouicience continued, for he also impregnated his second wife a second time. Curiously, he raised her two children, but not the other five.

The older of my two sisters mimicked my father in demeanor. She rarely smiled, and never praised anyone for anything sincerely. She was always austere. There was no familial troopbonding between any of us children.

My sister lived in competition with males. I remember her fighting boys, and winning. She seemed to be the defender of the family in my early years. She enjoyed argumentation, and often won.

Inexplicably to me, she rarely spoke a kind word to me. Her demeanor toward me was one of disgust and detestation. She'd look at me with contempt, but I didn't know why. Once I attempted to learn a card game. She appeared on the scene and commented that I had enough bad habits, and shouldn't play cards. I didn't know what a habit was, much less a bad habit.

Perhaps her resentment was engendered from having to babysit for me, her younger brother, in my infancy. Again, I had no choice.

Later, while visiting my sister, I observed that she treated her own children the same way. She'd scream at her daughter, "You're giving me a headache." I don't know how any of her children turned out.

The younger of my two sisters is similar to Connie, who became my mistress. She was the ideally feminine sister. Mostly, she grew up with the demeanor of a typical girl. She was friendly, and had a girl-friend. She was the one I strived to be close to, but she didn't let me.

My sisters argued and fought most of the time, and I don't remember them ever being friendly with each other. To my sisters, I was a pest. Since my mother took her frustrations out on me, my sisters followed the same pattern, especially since I was a male.

When my oldest sister went to college, the younger of the two sisters assumed dominance in the house. When my mother went to work, she became cook and babysitter. As my mother punished me, so did the younger of my two sisters. She ordered me around as though I were her own son. She beat me as though I were her child to punish. As I grew up, it never occurred to me to retaliate.

Her visage, demeanor, and morphology became imprinted uopn my developing lovemap. Her hairless vulva became imprinted upon my mind when I was as young as three years of age. Subsequently, forty years later, it was a girl much like her who would lead me into twenty-four eroticized armed robberies. Imprinting is a powerful force.

Once, after a failed romance when I was about twenty-one years of age, I drove to California to visit my sister, but she wouldn't let me stay at her home. She suggested that I find some girl to sleep with. I found several. Today, my sister won't even let me know my niece.

When I was about three years old, my neighbors had a little girl, my friend Pam, of the same age. She was an adorable little girl. My mother took photos of us sitting on a log in my backyard. I still remember snuggling next to Pam on that log to have our photos taken, as we smiled and held hands.

Pam and I observed that adults pressed their lips together to kiss. We enjoyed each other's playful company. Somehow we sensed that kissing should be done in private, so we hid under my back porch steps. Endearingly, we pressed our sensitive lips together, and liked it. In fact, I still recall the tenderness of that first reciprocal kiss. We were rehearsing our subsequent lover-lover pairbond, which would follow our puberty.

Meanwhile, and inopportunely, my spiteful sister discovered our innocent kissing. She ran directly to my perverse mother.

With severe words of admonishment, Pam was sent home. Her mother never allowed Pam to visit my backyard again. Our rehearsal kiss was considered evil, and unforgivable. But there was no evil in our kissing; there was only affection.

My mother scolded me for sharing an innocent kiss with my playmate. To my misinformed parents, I had committed an act worthy of punishment. Naturally, I had to atone for this sinful act of kissing, especially since the Holy Bible advocates beating a child to deliver it from some threatening hell.

Consequently, I was taken into my parents' bedroom to be spanked. My helpless body was placed over the side of my parents' bed. In my childhood mind, I hadn't done anything wrong. My father, who weighed about two hundred pounds, commenced beating my buttocks. The harsh blows to my incriminated body sent intense pain through me. I couldn't protect myself, nor could I expain my actions. My mother watched from the bedroom door as my small body was beaten, as tradition erroneously dictated.

Surprisingly, my penis swelled. Suddenly, an arcane metamorphosis occurred, turning the pain in my buttocks to a warm and euphoric feeling. I didn't know what was happening to me, but it felt good, and protective.

Vaguely, I recall my father saying to my mother, "Why is your son excited?" Euphemistically, excited meant being genitically aroused. Certainly, I question why he couldn't say, "Why is your son's penis erect?" Didn't he know it was engendered by child abuse?

Incidentally, today, my father denies this episode of our lives. Well, that's because this imprint didn't imprint on his developing lovemap, whereas it vandalized mine. Since I haven't spoken with my mother in twenty years, I don't know if she remembers it. Currently, my father suggests forgetting the past. "They were bad times," he says. If I could have discharged those childhood memories from my brain, I wouldn't be in prison.

I suppose that my parents thought I was born with a developed brain, and automatically knew correct behavior in this mutable world. So, instead of being trained in a viable behavior, I was labeled bad, scolded, and spanked. Also, if my inexperienced childhood behavior merited it, I was starved. I was forced into eating distasteful food with threats of being burned with a hot iron if I did not comply. My sisters reveled in my punishment.

Being born into a world of giants, otherwise known as parents, I needed my brain to protect me. Thus, when I went to bed without eating, my erotic brain provided me another realm within which to indulge. Contrary to psychiatric jargon, I didn't escape from reality. My brain devised imagery that actually existed as reality. My brain's imagery facilitated my actuality, especially since I lived in a punitively metaphorical hell. Punishment vandalized me.

Today, of necessity, I wear glasses. During the second grade I couldn't see the blackboard clearly. When I failed, I was verbally abused and spanked. When my myopic mother instructed me in arithmetic, I couldn't learn, for I dreaded being screamed at and spanked again. I was told that I was stupid. However, it was my parents who were at fault, not me.

Once I hid under the dining room table while my mother attacked my father with a rolling pin, and I watched in terror. They were fighting over an alleged infidelity of my father. I don't doubt my father's infidelity, especially since he still doesn't know what causes either his genital arousal or attraction to specific types of females. However, that acrimonious scene became imprinted upon and vandalized my developing lovemap.

Later, when my parents were living in marital separation, my mother taught me to hate my father. When he attempted to visit his coital mistakes, otherwise known as his children, my mother ordered me to throw stones at his jeep. In church, at the same age, and at home, I was told to honor my mother and my father. I never knew why.

The preceding incidents were imprinted upon my developing lovemap without my prepubertal consent. Small wonder that I and my sisters ended our first marriages in divorce.

Curiously, my mother abandoned me when I became the victim of her bipolar disorder, which I inherited. It was my father who came to my rescue.

There is a similarity between the paraphilia and the bipolar disorder. Both of them are episodic in their effect upon the victim's life. Also, they have a way of being in abeyance, thereby making the victims believe they're cured, but the symptoms always return. Whether you have a bipolar disorder or a paraphilia, you are always a victim.

My mother had the habit of wrapping her menstrual pads in toilet paper, then leaving them in the bathroom for a few days. I smelled something, which was similar to the odor of my mother. Although I didn't know exactly where the blood-soaked menstrual pads derived from, I guessed that they pertained to my mother's sexuality. Yet, whom would I question?

Consequently, that niche which lies between women's thighs became most alluring. Subsequently, peeking under the skirts of females became a preoccupation, and a source of religious guilt.

Now, and for the previous twenty years, I have been erotically excitable by smelling specific females during the menstrual period. However, I'm not dependent on feminine odor for genital arousal.

Paradoxically, today's television advertises menstrual hygiene products over every station, and in front of all age groups. I wonder what parents are telling their five-year-old sons as to where feminine hygiene products are used. Society wonders, and agonizes, as to why there is so much genital/sexual curiosity. It speaks of genitalia, but forbids the viewing of genitalia on television. Show murder and torture instead!

Typically foolish, my mother put me to bed before I was tired or ready. If I talked or moved too much in bed, my older sister or mother would beat me with a stick. The stinging of my skin was excruciating at first. Then an exhilaration permeated every cell of my childhood organism.

I didn't comprehend it then, but my erotic brain had mitigated the pain by inducing my genital/sexual arousal, transforming it into masochistic euphoria. Thus, my organism used my genital lust, which should have been coexistent with lovebonding after puberty, to facilitate my survival against my family abusers.

Frequently I would go to bed feeling an incitement to lower my pajama bottoms. Mental images of being beaten on my buttocks would traverse my mind. As I lowered my pajama bottoms, my penis would swell. The genital feeling was distractive and soothing. Then I'd lie on my erect penis and rub it against the sheet. The friction sensitized my penis and my mental imagery stimulated me, euphorically. Once I awoke lying on top of my blanket with my buttocks exposed. The only thing that I could remember was my erotic fantasy. Early in my life, buttocks and pain had become connected with genitals.

At about eleven years old, when it came time to take a bath, I'd be disposed to fill the bathtub with very hot water. An inclination for specific pain beckoned me to lower my buttocks into the hot water, then ignore the initial contact, which was excruciating. Once my penis swelled, the pain transformed into a euphoric warmth. My vandalized lovemap's lust facilitated a masochistic metamorphosis.

After my buttocks were bright red, I'd view them in the mirror. The image of red buttocks facilitated even more intense genital swelling, and even more pervasive erotic imagery. Then, by rubbing alcohol on my scalded buttocks, my masochistic euphoria would elevate. Actually, my entire organism felt as swollen as my penile engorgement. It was enrapturing.

My paraphilic fix also elevated when I strapped my buttocks with a belt. I'd lash my battered buttocks until my arm reached exhaustion. But it was such an ecstatic feeling that I couldn't want to cease.

I always had a dread of discovery. If my masochistic actions were discovered by my uninformed parents or my sneaky sisters, they would condemn me, and punish me more. Pardoxically, they were the very ones who had precipitated my developing masochism, however inadvertently. There was one occasion when the older of my two sisters poked her head into the bathroom to see what I was doing. But she never questioned me about it afterwards.

Paradoxically, when no one was home, I'd find the enema nozzle. Since I'd been given an excess of enemas, I developed an erotically distorted association with them. Thus, when I'd insert the enema nozzle into my anal canal, my penis would swell, accompanied by relevant mental imagery of someone receiving an enema, or the protrusion of young female bottocks.

It was the reflexive swelling of my penis that compelled me. I could not yet have an ejaculatory orgasm. Perhaps my erotic brain was rehearsing me for the future of penile orgasms under the sponsorship of a vandalized lovemap. Probably I was functioning under the aegis of a redesigning lovemap, as a sequal to infant vandalizing.

Occasionally I'd take several belts into the bathroom and wrap them around my thighs. I might have been twelve years old at that time. My erectile penis would be pressed between my thighs, and straining, causing intense erotic euphoria. Spontaneously, I'd imagine being restrained and spanked while in this eroticized position.

Compulsively, I'd utilize another belt to lash my exposed buttocks, while my penile erection was interfemorally restrained. I didn't want to cease strapping my sore buttocks. The induced erotic euphoria was so compelling that I could have died in masochistic metamorphosis, blissfully.

My schoolteachers seemed to dislike me because I smiled too much, and didn't talk enough. Later I learned that smiling elicits suspicion. I failed the second grade. That was the year before I was fitted with eyeglasses. I didn't fail because I was dumb. I failed because I was chagrined most of the time, and I couldn't see the blackboard clearly. Yet I didn't want to wear glasses. They were stigmatizing. They made me picked upon.

I had an aversion to intermale rivalry and fighting. I despised foul banter. I saw so much family fighting at home that it terrified me. I didn't associate with the boys at school. I didn't troopbond. That made me an outcast. In elementary school, other boys shunned girls, but I adored them. I thought they were pretty and sweet.

Typically boys thought it was cool to belch, fart, spit, and fight. I had no interest in those accomplishments. They were not my idea of what would make me a man. I knew that I was a male because my genitals were different from those of my sisters. I was labeled as shy, but I wasn't shy, I was diffident. I was continuously misconstrued. Perplexity prevailed.

One of my teachers looked like my father's second wife. During that class, I'd sense an irrepressible urge to draw female buttocks with strap marks on them. The mental imagery that induced me to make these drawings swelled my erectile penis under my desk. Yet, I didn't choose to draw sadomasochistically.

During my elementary school years I serviced a paper route. Delivering papers wasn't always easy, especially since I had to live up to my father's standards of what a paperboy should be. It was my only means of obtaining spending money. I didn't earn much, about three dollars per week. However, it gave me a feeling of accomplishment. Typically, I'd buy model cars and candy bars.

One day snow was inundating the city. My shoes were wet. My feet were freezing. My ears were so cold they were stinging. There was no shelter, nowhere to hide from the cold, and my hands were numb. Even the cars with chains had difficulty driving through the menacing snow.

On my route, I had to pick up additional papers. The wind was blowing. I knelt to pick up my new stack of papers. I strived to secure the papers in my carrying belt, but weariness overcame me. I dropped the papers, and the wind scattered them. I cursed the sky above, and the earth beneath me. Wearily, I trudged through the deep snow. The force of the wind made my walk home a defeat. My only prevailing thought was to get home and be warm again, but the memory of the undelivered papers nagged me.

I had no idea how much time elapsed before I arrived home. I entered the front door. There I encountered my agitated mother. She had a stick in her hand. Evidently people on the route had called. Without giving me a chance to speak, she beat my buttocks without mercy. She chased me into the bedroom with a battering of baleful blows.

Suddenly, the thing that most perplexed my childhood occurred again. My prepubertal penis swelled. The pain on my buttocks became a warm sensation, a metamorphosis that protected me from maternal abuse.

My mother ordered me to take my pants down so she could lash me more, on my bare skin and buttocks. I couldn't do that because of my erect penis. She supposed that I was disobeying her, so she whipped me more. I heard her screaming that I was lazy and irresponsible. I didn't deliver all the newspapers. My side of the story didn't matter.

A stimulative feeling pervaded my welted thighs and buttocks. My body didn't flinch from her pounding stick. I didn't want her to cease beating my transformed senses, yet I didn't want her to suspect my euphoria.

My mother and father were divorced at the time. But my mother made sure that my father got her distorted story: I was irresponsible and lazy. He still believes it today.

One time I longed for the thrill of having extra money to buy some model cars. I walked my paper route daily with this objective in my mind. In fact, the pervasive thought of accumulating money facilitated my work. Finally, I garnered nine dollars. I felt ecstatic with monetary excitement. My brother observed my fiscal happiness. I threw the dollar bills up into the air so they would fall on my head. Well, my brother thought this was irresponsible behavior. He told my mother that if I threw my money around, I shouldn't have it. She screamed at me for being so careless with money, and took it away. Then she commenced beating my buttocks and thighs. I still hate her for that. Subsequently, I never saved money again. That whipping imprinted upon my childhood mind a connection between money, pain from punishment, and females. I acquired a distorted sense of money connected with eroticism. For thirty years of my adult life, I would earn great amounts, only to spend it all on girls. Until I studied sexology, and learned of chrematistophilia, I didn't know why I had behaved that way.

When I observed my sisters having their buttocks cracked with a paddle or lashed with a strap, I was aquiver with tension in my penis. Thus, my developing lovemap connected penile sensations with punishment, and the spanking of female buttocks, but not with female genitalia.

My elementary school provided sex-education instruction—instruction in reproductive or genital function, that is. Nonetheless, my absurd mother prohibited my attendance. She kept me ignorant of my human sexuality, and that of the female. Little did she know of my masochistic erections, for which she herself was responsible.

Once, while my class was attending the euphemistically named sex-education classes, I visited the library. Two agemates sat in a corner with a book and giggled. I moved closer to see what was so funny. It was a nude statue of a female. I wondered why they were amused. I questioned my own lack of amusement, for I enjoyed the female form, however displayed. Somehow my mind resisted the vulgarizing of the female form.

Inquisitively, I searched the public libraries to discover my genital quandry. I needed to know why I experienced inopportune penile erections. I yearned to understand the genital difference between boys and girls. I longed to comprehend my attraction to girls in one way, but distance from them in other ways. Truly, I enjoyed girls, but didn't know how to pairbond with them. My lover-lover pairbonding was distorted and impaired even though I was still a child. It was how I viewed female and male interaction at home. Since my sisters expressed hatred toward me, my brain supposed that girls in general would behave the same way.

I often surprised my teachers. When I studied for a vocabulary test, I achieved the highest grade. Then I dreaded the attention of achievement because I'd blush. I enjoyed praise from the girls, but the blushing made me want to die. Yet I couldn't stop blushing any more than I could stop my penis from erecting when I was spanked. During the sixth grade, when I was becoming pubertal, my mental imagery was deluged with blushing, female buttocks, and spanking. I spent much of my time holding my erect penis through a hole in my pocket. I enjoyed learning, but my spontaneous erections distracted me. They impaired troopbonding with classmates, and pairbonding with girls.

Even in my neighborhood I didn't play male games which I considered insipid. Boys spent their time vying to prove who was tougher than the other. I couldn't imagine anything except being with neighborhood girls. Their parents forbade our friendship. Parents' concepts of human sexuality were so distorted that they made friendship with their daughters abnormal. They vandalized the pairbond between female and male. That impaired my pairbonding with females for the rest of my life. In an all-male prison, I have discovered that all inmates suffer from impaired female bonding as well as from distorted intermale bonding.

During the summer between the sixth and seventh grades, I suppose my pubertal life began. I entered the seventh grade with acne, muscle development, and an incessant penile erection. The girls in my class were no longer the opposite sex, they were erotic allurements. The composite imagery of my developed lovemap swelled my penis on sight of their hair, eyes, nose, mouth, neck, shoulders, breasts, arms, waists, hips, thighs, legs, and the sound of their feminine voices. I didn't understand it, nor was I rehearsed.

My intermale attachment with classmates was impaired and disturbing. I couldn't comprehend why the boys had to fight with each other, why they needed to use foul language to speak with one another, why they laughed about farting and belching, why a boy had to walk, talk, dress, spit, play ball, and act in a specific manner to be a man. Moreover, why did they speak of girls pejoratively? According to the boys in my class, school, and neighborhood, girls were whores, bitches, scags, sluts, weak, and less than any man. Conversely, I adored, cherished, and found the girls delicious, delectable, and delightful.

Whereas my boy-girl partnering was impaired, the other boys' girl-boy partnering was distorted. Unlike other boys, I never compared myself to the girls, either physically or behaviorally. Somehow, amid all the distortions of my childhood, I knew that I was male by virtue of my genitalia and nothing more, and that girls were female in view of their genitalia.

Erroneously, my mother, my sisters, and my church had taught me that my genitals are something to be ashamed of, especially in relation to girls. I didn't ever think of my erectile penis as being welcomed by girls. I didn't connect my penis with the vagina, either in coital fantasy or in actuality. Although I was genitally aroused much of the time, it never occurred to me that my penile swelling was in response to actual female images. Since my early childhood, my penile erections had been associated with punishment and spankings. I had often avoided female classmates. Mostly, I didn't want the girls to see my erect penis protruding through my trouser leg. Paradoxically, my sudden and overwhelming genital swelling impaired all possibility of affectionate pair-bonding with a girl.

My misguided mother and cruel sisters had been wrong about heterosexual love and lust. My first year in the seventh grade elicited more erotic attention from female classmates. Moreover, one particular female classmate found me irresistibly attractive, and she wasn't repulsed by my penis. She was Betty, an ideally pretty blonde, with a precociously well proportioned body. While walking between classes, I'd gaze at Betty's pear-shaped buttocks. Then I'd conceal my raging penis with my school books. Although I didn't know it, Betty found my genital arousal for her inviting, not repulsive. Unfortunately, when she flirted with me all I did was blush.

Betty and I attended the same art class. Frequently, I'd catch myself staring at her nubile body. I worried that she might notice my stares. It was the form of her hipline and buttocks that tormented me. Now I know that all male primates stare—eye contact is just the beginning, and it's essential. Otherwise nothing happens.

One day my art teacher sent me to the art supply room alone. Shortly thereafter, Betty opened the door. Her demeanor was randy. Alas, I was unrehearsed for heterosexual love and lust. Betty approached me audaciously and gazed into my eyes. My penile erection was ready, but I wasn't. The indoctrination of my childhood made me feel uncomfortable and embarrassed, whereas I should have felt the joy of pairbonded love and lust. No one at home had ever praised me for my postpubertal manhood. I didn't know that I was alluring to girls.

Betty and I were standing next to an empty table. Betty climbed onto the table seating herself on the edge of it. While seating myself next to her, I tried to disguise the hardness of my penis. Then Betty tugged her black skirt up to her hips. When I observed her smooth thighs and white panties, fluid from my penis oozed onto my leg. Betty knew what she wanted, and probably guessed that I was not experienced with girls romantically. She encouraged me by unbuttoning her white blouse. Her breasts were luring. I couldn't be appropriately lured.

Putting her lips to my neck, Betty kissed me. Although she encouraged my lustful reciprocation, I remained immobile. Within my mind I agonized, for I didn't know why I couldn't reciprocate. At three years of age, I had been punished for sharing an innocent kiss with Pam, my playmate, which would have been a rehearsal for that day with Betty. I didn't want to reject Betty, but the vandalization of that kiss in childhood had begun the vandalization of my lovemap into the cartography of masochism. Betty's warm, sensual body, and her eagerness to be with me didn't stir my lips, hands, or penis to a repeat of that disaster. I could not reciprocate lustfully.

Then, her love and lust shunned, Betty withdrew her physical affection and jumped to the floor. With a dejected look on her face, she ran to the door. Jumping from the table, I grabbed her, but hesitantly. Angrily, Betty screamed for me to release her. For the few seconds that I held her body next to me, I realized the wonderful feeling of heterosexual lust. I released Betty, and when the door closed behind her, I knew that it was too late. I cried.

Her erotic affection for me was dispelled forever. Betty didn't speak to me from that day forth. Consequently, I wanted to die. I cursed the sky above and the earth beneath me. It seemed as though I was being punished again for desiring feminine affection.

School and neighborhood boys were participating in baseball, basketball, soccer, track, and other stereotypical male sports. I played some catch football, but my mother didn't like the boys I played with. Nonetheless, my teenaged body was full of untapped power.

One year, for my birthday, my mother's boyfriend gave me a set of barbells. Arriving home from school each day, I'd enjoy a workout with my heavy weights. My physique developed to be strong and muscular. Nonetheless, my mother and my sisters wouldn't give me credit for my masculinity. They didn't want their praiseworthy comments to swell my head, though that's what I needed. As a result, I did not understand that my muscular body was a lure for many girls.

My weightlifting elicited intermale competition. Unfortunately, my gender role was not that of typical boys. I couldn't force myself to belittle girls in banter, or vulgarize them in any fashion. Therefore, I wasn't accepted as one of the boys. To me, possessing excess muscle didn't make me better than a girl, but to typical teenaged boys it did.

I owned the power and reflexes to defeat most school boys. I was typecast as a weakling, for I had developed an aversion to fighting. It was a result of watching my mother and father along with my two sisters indulge combatively since my early childhood. It seemed illogical to be hostile. Life was hell for me.

During my early teenaged years, I experienced an uncannily irresistible urge to dress in certain pieces of my mother's clothing. It was not her clothing I sought, it was how I'd look with her clothing on. When no one was home, I'd select specific pieces of her clothing to wear. Her girdle was first, for it concealed and restrained my erected penis. The encasement of my penis engendered a compressed eroticized energy.

The mirror in my mother's bedroom facilitated the viewing of myself as a masqueraded female. Although the mirrored image was not me, it exhibited the clothed form of a young female. An hour might have passed while I was adoring the mirrored impostor of myself. Frequently, I'd expose the buttocks of the mirrored girl. Genital lust elevated as the actual scene paralleled my imagery. Nonetheless, I never had longed to be a female, nor did I have any inclination to appear in public as a male in female clothing.

Finally, that scenario of being cross dressed consummated in my masqueraded self being spanked. I didn't spank myself, I spanked the buttocks of the girl, as reflected in my mother's bedroom mirror. To inflict optimal pain, I beat her/my buttocks with a wooden stick or extension cord. That lashing or beating continued until my arm reached exhaustion. Then, with my/her omnipresent sadomasochism, I'd achieve an exhilarating orgasm. It felt too good to be wrong.

Irrespective of where I went, what I did, or with whom I was, mental imagery disposed me to spank myself, especially to facilitate optimal orgasms. So I'd strive to be alone at home as often as possible. My penis was persistently in a semierect state, and always there was masochistic imagery and ideation.

Arriving home from junior high school, I would rush to my bedroom, where I would remove my trousers. While lying on my bed, I'd beat my bare buttocks. My penile erection was squeezed between my thighs and oozing. Longingly, I'd wish that a girl could spank me, for I couldn't spank myself fiercely enough. While paddling my buttocks, fluid flowed from my penis onto the sheet. My penis seemed as hard as wood.

My imagined scenes were mostly of beaten buttocks. Rarely did my paraphilic imagery reflect actual persons in detail, only bodily parts. While my self-inflicted punishment prevailed, the dread of discovery disturbed me; I yearned to admit my masochism, and perhaps be saved from my internal tyrant. To whom might I report my paraphilia without condemnation? There was no one.

During classroom periods, I held or fondled my semierect penis through the hole in my pocket nearly all day. Although I strived to, I couldn't concentrate on school work. I was preoccupied with finding a place to spank myself and achieve orgasm.

Occasionally, while seated on my front porch, I'd watch a cute blonde walk by my house on her way to or from somewhere. I wanted to speak with her. My penis swelled as I watched her. I discovered her name to be Darlene. One day I met her walking home from school. She was a sweet and pretty girl, but my penile lust embarrassed me, and my relationship with her was impaired. Arriving at my house, I'd conceal my swollen erection with my books while we stopped to talk. After Darlene had departed, I found my mother watching me from behind the front door of my home. She warned me to keep away from girls like Darlene. When I questioned my mother about her criticism, she labeled Darlene a "hussy." My mother didn't know anything about Darlene's sexual behavior. My mother condemned all manifest heterosexuality.

While walking through the halls at school, I'd often hear a girl's voice utter, "Hi handsome." I could only blush. Later, I discovered who my elusive admirers were, but I couldn't reciprocate their interest. Little did I realize it then, but many schoolgirls would have accommodated my penile lust, and there was no need to hide my genital arousal from girls who expressed an eroticized interest in me. No one ever taught me that love and lust should coexist in the pairbonding of female and male. Moreover, no one knew how to define heterosexual love in order to teach me. In my youth, genital lust was utterly disowned, though babies were still conceived.

My mother was suspicious of everyone. She resisted the signs of heterosexuality in her children. However, my sisters and I were maturing along with our interest in heterosexual love and lust. At the time, I was about fourteen with one sister two years older and another sister six years older.

On one occasion of suspicion, my sister, who was an ideally pretty sixteen-year-old, was seated on our front porch. I sat nearby. Several of the boys who lived in our neighborhood were visiting my sister. She apparently reveled in their attention. Suddenly and intrusively, my mother stormed onto the front porch from the house. She grabbed my sister by the hair, pulling her into the house. I overheard my mother yelling, "That's like a bunch of dogs hanging around a bitch in heat." The boys were surprised by my mother's rudeness and departed shaking their heads. I overheard my mother and sister quarreling with each other for the next hour.

On another occasion, my sister had an evening date with a man. While waiting for the two of them to arrive on the porch after their date, my mother paced the floor forebodingly. They returned. Just before departing, the man kissed my sister near the front door. From behind the door, my mother interrupted their kiss and pulled my sister into our house. She rudely dismissed my sister's date, and quarreled with her over a kiss. What's wrong with kissing a girl good night, I wondered? Consequently, my mother debased my perception of heterosexual kissing.

Distortions about my heterosexuality continued. For example, my father left home for another woman, and my mother sought privacy with men in her bedroom. So it seemed proper for me to pursue another boy's girlfriend.

A girl named Gail who lived in my neighborhood visited an age-mate who lived nearby. She entranced me with her nubile physique and long brown hair. The distant sound of her voice excited me. I longed to walk, talk, and gaze at her. The fact that she was another boy's girlfriend somehow enticed me. In fact, secrecy was a significant part of erotic partnerships in my childhood.

On one warm summer day, I walked with Gail to an unoccupied church. While inside the church, she was coaxing me, but I couldn't reciprocate affectionately or lustfully. Although I think she knew, I didn't want her to know that my penis was erect. She felt rejected and I felt ashamed of my genital arousal.

Several days later, Gail asked me why I didn't kiss her while we were in the church. "You could have taken my panties down if you wanted," she said. I didn't know how to reply. I didn't realize that it was normal for girls and boys to share their lustfulness. I was mostly perplexed. I still couldn't perform like a boy in love with a girl. In short, since my penis swelled when I was spanked, I wasn't sure why it swelled with a girl. And there was no one to ask for enlightenment.

On the one hand, my mother disowned her involvement in lust with other men. On the other hand, she gave birth to two baby boys about ten to twelve years after my birth. When questioned twenty years after their birth, my father disowned one of them. No one talked about it. It just happened.

Meanwhile, my two sisters went to college. Since my mother worked to support my younger brothers and me, I was charged with caring for my brothers. I discovered cooking, washing clothes, housekeeping, and child care. My brothers were as poorly informed about their sexuality and heterosexuality as I was.

Not too far away there lived a teenaged girl, Laura. Her parents owned a swimming pool. One day Laura's mother, my mother, my two brothers, and Laura and I were swimming in the pool. Later, everyone vacated the pool, except Laura and me. When I touched her tender skin, my penis swelled. I couldn't make it deflate. When I climbed out of the pool, my erection protruded through my swimming suit. Laura's mother was enraged at the sight of my erect penis in the proximity of her daughter. Consequently, I was barred from their pool, and never allowed to be near Laura again.

For the second time in my life a girl was taken from me, and again it was not for anything malicious. Erroneously, I learned that my penile erection was not to be shared with females. This made more hell in my life.

My last year of school was in the tenth grade. Achieving orgasms preoccupied me five or six times per day. As my eyes viewed the girls who were in my class and in the halls of the school, my penis swelled in response. My mental pictures were of buttocks being spanked, and of specified girls whom I observed. But I never imaged coital activity with any girl.

After school, I attended the YMCA to work out with barbells. I knew little to nothing about male homosexuality. Nonetheless, I observed men staring at me while I showered. In fact, men were repulsive to me, so I stopped attending the YMCA.

At eighteen years of age, I enlisted in the U.S. Army. My enlistment in the army was a coping strategy. I longed to escape the domination of my mother along with her misguided attitude toward life. In my ignorance of paraphilias, I assumed that I could change the masochized imagery and ideation of my mind. I had to do something, and the army seemed a place to start.

During the first two months in the army, I applied for the General Educational Development examination. A preliminary course of seven weeks was required to prepare for the GED test. Before the course commenced, a major inquired about my schooling, for my Army Entrance Examination score indicated a second year college level. The major suggested that I take the test immediately. I took the GED and passed it. My accomplishment surprised me, for my family had declared me stupid. Subsequently, I aimed for self-improvement.

My basic training in the army was easy, for my body was in excellent physical shape. Although I had nothing to worry about, I experienced recurrent depression, which perplexed me greatly. Unfortunately, I didn't get along any better with the other privates than I did with the boys at home. I couldn't understand why the other privates thought it necessary to speak vulgarly, particularly in reference to women.

With my army uniform on, I elicited the attention of many women, but I lacked coital experience. Therefore, I sought the services of a prostitute to experience genital union for the first time. It seemed appropriate to copulate with a prostitute, for my penis and the prostitute were both condemned by society, although I didn't understand why.

I met a hooker named Mona. I felt comfortable with her so I admitted my virginity. Somehow I sensed that Mona deserved money for copulating with me. I didn't assume that I was buying sexual favors. Nonetheless, Mona and I indulged coitally, but I was not delighted. My disappointment was not her fault, for she was affectionate and willing to please me. Mona had no way of knowing that my orgasms were masochized, nor did she know what spurred me to lust with her.

By copulating with Mona, I dispatched the stigma of not having any sex. Privately, I longed to find a prostitute who would spank me. In short, Mona was the first, but by no means the last, of a magnitude of hookers I sought to facilitate my orgasms.

During my second eight weeks of military training, I was stationed at Fort McClellan, Alabama. At that time, Fort McClellan was the home for a Women's Army Corps detachment. There were three thousand women on my base. I was outnumbered by one hundred women to one man.

Nightly I attended the Army Service Center and danced with dozens of the female privates. Nightly, my erectile penis swelled and poured fluid onto the leg of my uniform. Testicular pain waxed so intensely that I could barely walk back to my barracks. My penis rarely deflated, which forced me to live with an aching scrotum.

Eventually I met a WAC named Lynda who said that she was in love with me. She assumed that I'd be sexually assertive with her, and was disappointed when I failed to kiss her. Nonetheless, Lynda kissed me, and for the first time in my eighteen years of life, kissing was good. My masochism seemed outside of my partnership with Lynda, but something impaired my partnership with her anyhow. As much as I yearned to explore her naked body something held me back. My lust was active betweeen my legs and in my mind, but I couldn't share it with her. Something impaired my lovebonding, but I didn't know what it was, nor did I know whom to ask.

The other privates returned to the barracks boasting of their penile conquests. Although I'm sure many of them were exaggerating, I couldn't copulate with a girl who wanted me to copulate with her. Consequently, I failed my tests at Fort McClellan. I wanted to die.

After five months in the army, I received orders to go to Germany, following a sixty-day leave. Lynda and I exchanged addresses and final words of affection, but we never spoke again.

Arriving back in Baltimore from Fort McClellan, I discovered that my mother had moved and remarried. It appeared to have been a marriage of convenience, not involving the state of love. Since I was leaving the United States for over two years, my mother treated me to a vacation in Ocean City, Maryland.

Swimming daily in the salt water and being tanned by the sun had healing effects on my acned skin. My muscular body was quite impressive, but I didn't exhibit the assertive demeanor that usually accompanied a muscular physique. Nonetheless, the girls on the beach were inclined toward me, and my penis swelled. But I still didn't know why it swelled.

A voluptuous teenaged girl flirted with me: Eve. There I was with another beautiful woman, but my pairbonding was still impaired. When I walked along the beach with her, my genitals swelled and ached. My unassertive lustfulness vexed me, and probably made her feel undesirable. In fact, her genital arousal wasn't even considered by me. I didn't know what was wrong with me. I longed anew for death.

After three weeks with Eve, we exchanged addresses. We left Ocean City. I returned to Baltimore to continue my military leave. Eve returned to Virginia and promised to write when she got home. My mother mocked my romantic affairs, saying that I was foolish. She didn't give me credit for being a healthy male. To her, I couldn't possibly be in love, particularly since she didn't know anything about being in love.

Shortly before my leave ended, I walked with Gail, the girl I didn't kiss in church, to a bus stop. By knowledge of hindsight, I was in love with her. At the bus stop Gail asked me for a quarter, which I gave to her. I think she kept that quarter in remembrance of me. Furthermore, she promised to write to me while I was stationed in Germany. I yearned to depart for Germany just to receive a letter from her.

Darlene, the girl my mother called a hussy, also gave me her address, asking that I write when I arrived in Germany. Contrary to what ignorant people think about me today, available girls were never a problem of mine. In fact, both Gail and Darlene were seeing other boys when I encountered them. And both of them preferred being with me. Moreover, I rejoiced in distracting the girls from the other boys.

I experienced masturbatory imagery of both Gail and Darlene. However, none of my mental scenes with those girls involved coital activity. I imaged their vulva or buttocks while I masturbated. Interestingly, their genitals were imagined hairless, although I had never seen them in actuality.

Since I would be in Germany for twenty-six months, I visited a relative (my unofficial stepfather's mother) during my last week in America. I was riding my bike and thinking about the forthcoming years in a foreign country when I encountered two girls riding their bikes. Their teenaged bodies induced engorgement of my penis immediately. There was no prior thought of genital arousal. My penis inflated like a balloon with the pressure of air being forced into it. Again, I was spellbound.

Both of the girls were wearing skimpy shorts and halter tops. I was new in their neighborhood so they asked me where I was from. After telling them about myself, they invited me to lunch. They didn't conceal their erotic inclination for me. Although I was genitally aroused, I had no impetus to copulate with either one of them. Nonetheless, they lured me with their erotic parts.

I don't know whose house we stopped at. One girl asked the other girl, "Are you going to bed with him?" Instead of those words thrilling me with lustful ideas, their coital interest in me caused despair. Meanwhile, my penile fluid dripped down the leg of my pants. In frustrating situations, my mother said, "I wish the world would end." I followed her example by internally wishing that I could die. I didn't know how to accept the lust or love of a woman.

The night before departing for Germany, I walked up and down Baltimore's Block. I found myself seeking the magazines of masochistic erotica. It frustrated me, for I didn't like those inclinations in myself. I longed to leave America, hoping that might make them go away.

It was August 1961 when I boarded the troop carrier departing for Germany. During fourteen weary days at sea, I read the Holy Bible. I read the Holy Bible as a coping tactic, for my life vexed me greatly. The Scriptures ostensibly offered me hopefulness, but I'd never met anyone who had benefited from the Scriptures.

After settling in at Taylor Barracks, Christianized religion played a daily role in my attitude toward life. The Christian God was supposed to be the source of love, though I had no concept of love's meaning. There seemed to be more than one meaning of the word love. Nonetheless, I felt optimistic, for my masochism was inactive.

Attending the chapel on my base were missionaries to servicemen who were associated with the Navigators. The Navigator I met taught me a unique method of memory and I applied it to memorizing Scriptures. I also involved myself in Bible study courses from the Moody Bible Institute. My active mind seemed to have no limitations. Within the first year of my study and memory work, I had memorized the New Testament. I thought that I was in control of my life, finally.

I had been involved in a Lutheran church during my childhood, but I didn't experience the subjective phenomenon of being born again until my scriptural studies in Germany. It was similar to the afterglow of an orgasm. I wondered about that interconnection.

Almost all of my orgasms within the first of my two years in Germany were the result of wet dreams. Although I don't recall the mental pictures that accompanied those nocturnal orgasms, I know they lacked genital interaction. Female imagery aroused me genitally, but not to copulate.

I was a student of the Navigators for a year when they invited me to a religious retreat. It was held at the General Walker Hotel in the Alps. The young maids at the hotel were most alluring. I sensed their actual form impinge upon my mind, but I couldn't stop it. As a result, my mind devised scenes suited to arouse me and facilitate orgasms. Turning to God's word, I prayed that those lustful images wouldn't overcome me and override my Christianity.

Nightly I strived to resist the eroticized and paraphilic images within my Christianized mind and body. Without my Christian consent, my mental scenes were of buttocks being spanked. My masochism had been evoked. The transformation was again like that of Dr. Jekyll turning into Mr. Hyde. An arcane circuit seemed to connect my brain with my genitals; I knew what was next.

One day that week,I took a walk in a nearby wooded area. I sought God's help in resisting the foreboding ritual of my own masochized lovemap. When my paraphilia is active, my perception is intense. Inanimate objects seemed animate, especially the sticks on the trees.

My interior and exterior monologue sounded the word—no! I imaged myself being whipped with a stick, and my erect penis swelled according. Newly devised scenes of female buttocks were extended for a spanking on my mental stage. My God failed me.

Kneeling under the trees, I released my swollen penis. Mysteriously, my fingers grasped a sturdy stick to beat my buttocks. With my pants down to my knees, which were bent on the dry leaves, I commenced whipping my bare buttocks. My penile fluid dripped onto the leaves. I strained to strike my buttock flesh as harshly as my arm would allow. My pulse rate increased. My skin began to perspire, soaking my shirt. I was angry with myself because my arm didn't strike my red rump fiercely enough.

I paused to observe my surroundings, especially to detect any observers. The pain was transforming into ecstasy in stages. So I returned to beating my buttocks to achieve masochistic euphoria. When I can strike my buttocks with no aversive sensation, the transformation is complete.

My mind and body achieved an ultimate high. My entire organism was stupefied. I wanted my euphoria to prevail forever. The metaphorical Mr. Hyde of my paraphilic lust had emerged and won. It felt absolutely wonderful. I couldn't believe that something so distorted could feel so good. My body fell onto the leaves in a state of orgasmic frenzy.

Afterward those who spoke with me thought that I had had a divine experience.

Christianity had a fail-safe mechanism. God can't be blamed for the individual's lack of faith. Therefore, I assumed that there was a deficiency in my belief, which accounted for God's failure to save me from masochism. Of course, it never occurred to me at that time that the reason for God's lack of help was that there is no God.

I wanted to be the ideal concept of normal, though I didn't really know what a normal person thought. I wondered about the private sexuality of others, and how many other people concealed sexual disorders. I had read about some religious leaders who did flagellate themselves. I didn't understand their reasons. I longed to purge this enemy from within, but revealing it might be worse than concealing it. Besides, how do I say, "I spank myself," without embarrassment and incrimination?

For the remainder of my tour of duty in Germany, I memorized the Holy Bible. Studying the word of God distracted me from my masochized imagery, but it didn't replace it. Discovering the Holy Bible raised a question that I couldn't answer: "Why did God condemn all future humans for the error of the two original humans?" Furthermore, I never heard anyone qualify the usage of the word love, and the Bible had three different meanings for it.

My father said he loved me, but abandoned me. My mother said she loved me, but beat and punished me. My God said he loved me, but failed me. My confusion about love endured.

Thirty days before returning to the United States, everyone in my company attended a reenlistment meeting. All but me. I accepted my honorable discharge and returned home. I was glad to be discharged from the army. Soldiers joking about women and degrading their femininity had become intolerable.

At home, I spoke with a local minister about attending his church's seminary. He was impressed with my Biblical knowledge. Taking the entrance examination to the seminary required two years of college, which I didn't have. I was allowed to take the test with the promise of entrance if I passed, and I passed.

I used the money I had saved during my time in the army to pay my tuition. Intellectually the seminary was not difficult. However, my masochized mental pictures and genital arousal recurred wtih increasing intrusiveness. Covertly, I discovered the masturbatory practices of some seminary students. None of those to whom I spoke could understand why God had made us disown our sexuality. I was an outstanding Christian externally, but internally I failed. Therefore, I departed from the seminary, and disengaged from the Christianized concept of God.

I returned home, but I didn't like it. Life held no meaning for me. I longed still for death. In my despair, I phoned Gail. Gail was delighted to hear from me. In fact, she'd been thinking about me prior to my phone call. My genitals swelled the second I heard her voice.

I couldn't talk, walk, look, or hear without genital arousal. The mere sound of Gail's voice swelled my penis, although we'd had no communication for twenty-six months. My voice impinged upon her in the same way. She admitted her horniness. We planned a meeting at Towson State College during the next day. While I was dressing for our assignation, my penis swelled in remembrance of Gail's physique. So I wore an athletic supporter to restrain my protruding erection.

If only I knew then what I know now about love and lust. The neighborhood girl I had left two years previously was the most beautiful girl on the college campus. Gail was strikingly appealing to me. During the twenty-four hours before meeting her, my mental stage rehearsed our encounter. I wasn't spanked by her during that intracranial rehearsal, but I wasn't copulated by her either. Just looking at her spurred me to a permeating lustiness. My athletic supporter was soaking wet, but I hadn't touched my genitalia.

Gail smiled and led me to the college chapel. I discovered that many students indulged their sexual appetites in the chapel. Gail pressed her lips to mine without hesitation. I was wtih a woman who didn't hesitate, but I was hesitating, though I didn't know why. I didn't need to pay her a sexual fee, but somehow I would have felt better if I did.

My right hand probed the front of Gail's sweater, but it was Gail who raised her sweater and unhooked her bra. Passionately, my mouth fixed itself to her breasts and sucked them fervently. I felt her hand tugging at my zipper, but I didn't release my raging penis. My foreplay was impaired, but there wasn't anything at the location or within Gail to stop me. My mind and body were in a state of eroticized frenzy.

We didn't copulate, but that was my doing. Something had impeded my assertiveness with a willing partner. It wasn't masochism this time. With the knowledge of hindsight, I know that my erotic partnership with girls had been impaired at three years of age. Yes, when my sister had tattled that she saw Pam and me kiss under the porch my girl and boy partnering had been impaired forever. Thereafter, it made me feel guilty about touching any girl, even one who wanted me to touch her.

Believe me, I wish my father had been so impaired with my mother. Perhaps I wouldn't be writing these diappointing words. I couldn't explain my behavioral sex impairment to Gail. She felt rejected, I assume. No, I couldn't discuss it with her. Now I wish that I could go back in time. I was in love with her. I am not accountable for my childhood. I was born into hell.

The first job of my adult life was in door-to-door sales. I liked the work because it kept me in visual contact with women. Moreover, the women to whom I sold products also liked me. In fact, many women within my territory requested, through the main office, that I remain their salesman. The female customers within my selling territory represented my own nonerotic harem.

Eventually, I discovered the many daughters of the women to whom I sold household products. Then I met a teenaged girl whose image reciprocated the composite images of my lovemap. Sharon was in her final year of high school. We started dating, but her mother didn't like my being Sharon's boyfriend. Her mother typecast me into a role I didn't fit. She claimed that her daughter should date boys from school, not men who were out of school and working. That complaint didn't stop us, for Sharon was inclined toward older men, and I was inclined toward younger women.

I thought that I was in love because my genitalia swelled in proximity to or fantasy about her. Normally, overstimulation meant masochistic behavior, but not with Sharon. I longed to tug her panties down, unsnap her bra, fondle and suck her nipples, but not be spanked by her. Our pairbond was fraught with discord, especially since I couldn't keep my hands and mouth off of her body. Unfortunately, I didn't understand my own genital arousal or hers.

My overarousal drove me mad. For me, there was no such cure as a cold shower. After my erectile penis swelled an orgasm had to follow. Otherwise, my scrotum and testicles would inflict an immobilizing pain within my groin. It was irrepressible, and irrespective of my choice. My love and lust were imbalanced, but I didn't know what to do about it.

During that period of my life, I experienced conflicts with my mother, and I had unresolved doubts about the existence of God. Consequently, I felt suicidal, particularly since Sharon's mother didn't want us dating. It would have helped if I'd known that I was a manic-depressive.

Sharon's mother spanked her three daughters. With me, Sharon once behaved in a way that merited a spanking—so I draped her across my lap and spanked her. Along with swelling my own genitals, Sharon was genitally aroused also. She reported other incidents whereby she became genitally aroused by a smack on her buttocks, and my maso-chism emerged again. When Sharon's mother observed her daughter's buttocks, she refused to allow us to date ever again.

Naturally, like any other couple who think they're in love, we met each other covertly. Sharon missed school to be with me, and she climbed out of her bedroom window to be with me. Those tactics didn't last, however.

Everyone told me there are a million other girls in the world. They suggested that I stop burning a torch for Sharon. They didn't know that every girl with long, auburn hair distracts me. Imagery of Shar-on's hips, thighs, breasts, and face inhabited my daydreams, irresistibly. At night I couldn't sleep without her pervading my dreams. I couldn't work and concentrate for any length of time without images of her inhabiting me. Blood surged into my penis whenever a vivid image of her voice was uttered on my mental stage. I couldn't cope.

As a result, I found myself persistently yearning for death. Although I had a new car, the sky was clear, I had money in my pocket, and I had no visible impairments, I felt like dying. It wasn't a choice, though. Ideation and mentation of suicide inhabited part of my brain.

I'd eat food for the taste of it, but not because I was hungry. I didn't even know what I ate after I ate it. Mostly, I didn't eat. I drank alcohol, but not because it tasted good. I consumed the alcohol to soothe the raging forces within me. Nothing helped.

Then, bless those little pills! If I ingested the right pills, I'd find temporary peace. I longed to sleep undisturbed for a while. Living had become intolerable. I found it difficult to endure a single day. I was irascible, but I didn't know why. The pills calmed me so I wasn't so irritable. I needed something to help me, for I couldn't help myself.

I couldn't go on living in the throes of mental agony. Thoughts of killing myself inhabited my mind and brain relentlessly. So I located the name of a psychiatrist in Silver Spring, Maryland. I made an appointment, and visited him one afternoon. I told him my story. My brain's talk was encouraging me to commit suicide, I reported. I found it onerous to survive one hour of life. Did he have a cure? He didn't have an instant cure, so I departed his office disappointed.

Subsequently, I visited the family doctor and asked him for sleeping pills. Not aware of my anguished mental state, he prescribed them for me. The only way to deal with this tormented mind was to kill the whole body, I assumed. However, I didn't really want to die.

Paradoxically, my orgasm was good, but everything accompanying it was bad. Once my lust started, I couldn't turn it off. I achieved erections, but I didn't know why. After five or six orgasms, I was still horny. What was wrong? I needed to find the state of love, but without my distorted lust.

I adored the many women of my life. I had affectionate bonds with some of them, and lustful attachments with the others. I couldn't get enough of them. I yearned to suck their breasts until I fell asleep. Genital unrest prevailed—orgasm after orgasm, but I couldn't be satisfied. I needed to snuggle without my penile lust.

I filled my prescription for sleeping pills. A reluctant tear rolled down my cheek as I considered leaving the girls I knew as friends. I examined the little bottle of red pills. I didn't really want to die. I simply couldn't go on living this way. Death seemed the only tenable solution. My enemy inhabited me, so where could I hide?

Paula was one of the girls with whom I had a nonerotic pairbond. I informed her of my despair over the telephone. Although she did not seek to rescue me, and I did not seek her condolence, Paula expressed a magnitude of compassion, and I relished that. She said goodbye, as though she believed my fatal intentions. My affection for her incited that final goodbye.

Gail panicked when I disclosed my despair and suicidal intent. She strived to discourage my ingestion of the sleeping pills. I adored her, but she didn't understand. When my erect penis swelled while speaking with Gail, I couldn't live any longer. I hung up the telephone and carried the bottle of sleeping pills to my car.

I swallowed every pill. I was parked in a lot full of shoppers. Driving my car until I crashed was my aim, but the effect of the sleeping pills dulled my reflexes. Reclining on my car seat, I felt peace within my mind and body. My goal was achieved. My own lust was deprived of another victory. The love I sought no longer mattered.

Instead of dying, I slept for three days. I later learned that Gail had called my mother, concerned over my suicidal intention. My body was delivered to a hospital, where the medical staff saved my life. Why couldn't they have said, "Let this man die in peace"? When I awoke in the hospital, a police officer informed me that attempting suicide is a criminal offense. No respect for my anguish! When the charges were dropped, in my immobilized state, a thought occurred to me: I can't live, and now I'm told that I can't die.

No one in my family showed any empathy. What drove me to suicide didn't enter anyone's mind. My mother visited me to disown me, for I had disgraced her. She didn't consider that she might be the source of my bipolar and sexual disorder. My mother never considered that her mood swings were caused by a disorder, and that I had inherited it from her. Since my mother didn't want any of her own children, her opportune disownment of me didn't seem too strange to me.

While I was recuperating, a nurse chastized me. She said, "You're in good physical condition, so why would you attempt to kill yourself? There are patients who want to live, but can't." I didn't know how to reply. Her insensitive comment perplexed me. Although I didn't need condolence, I needed help.

Not knowing any better, my mother signed me into a mental hospital. The doctors spoke with me only occasionally, and concluded that my suicidal attempt was over love. Lovesickness, I called it. Sharon was foremost on my mind, but she wasn't accountable for my despair. I realized how doctors and nurses could be myopic. I should have spoken up, but I didn't know how to explain myself.

Paula visited me. She was glad that I didn't die. She asked me to visit her after leaving the hospital. One visiting day, Sharon arrived. Every nerve in my body became frenzied. My penile lust was instantly activated. I longed to speak with her without my genital urgency protruding from between my legs. Alone with her, I couldn't resist the urge to grasp her jutting breasts. I yearned to bandy words of affection with her, but my lust reacted to her sexy body instead.

On another day, my father surprised me with a visit. Other than Paula, he was the only person to express sympathy. My father couldn't empathize however, for he'd been injured in combat, and struggled to live. Also, he'd observed critically wounded soldiers who still longed to live. He uttered words of encouragement. After a month, my father arranged for my release from the hospital.

It seemed as though I was back where I started. I was in a quandary. Emphatically, I hated life and all that it stood for. My self was divided.

Like most troubled people, I thought I could run from my problems. I drove to California. Although I didn't know it then, I was in one of the manic phases of my bipolar disorder, which facilitated my driving from Maryland to California in fifty hours. Ignorantly, I assumed that I could escape that which inhabited my mind and body.

Upon arriving in Santa Monica, I attempted to telephone my sister, the one who had vandalized me as a child. Somehow I dialed the wrong number. Instead, I phoned a girl who became curious about me. Several hours later we met. Since I didn't have much money, she bought dinner for me. There I was, three thousand miles from my home, and I'm with a girl. Of course, being a salesman, I'd learned to communicate verbally quite well. Although I didn't appreciate it, most girls considered me quite handsome.

By late evening, the California girl and I were together. She expected me to kiss, fondle, and copulate with her. I always failed to associate my genital arousal with a girl's vagina, but with spanking. I suppose she was surprised and thought that she was not erotically desirable. She invited me to sleep at her apartment that night.

The next day I searched for a job. I needed money. I got a job at a car wash after I explained my homeless situation. Then I found a cheap motel to stay at. I learned about life the hard way.

Eventually, I visited my West Coast sister. I wasn't welcomed as her brother, nor did her husband want me sleeping at their home. I departed quite disappointed even though this sister had treated me with condescension throughout my childhood. She'd become an idealist, and from what I hear she still is idealistic. That visit occurred twenty-five years ago, and I haven't seen her since.

Retrospectively, I can recall an incident of this sister's insensitivity and cruelty. Shortly after my second set of teeth grew in, one of them was accidentally broken. The nerve of the tooth was exposed, leaving me in much pain. Well, with reluctance, my mother charged my sister with the task of escorting me to the dentist. My mother concerned herself with the expense of the dentist, not my painful mouth. When the dentist pulled out my tooth, I traveled home with my sister. My mouth was in pain. I couldn't resist crying. But my sister demanded that I shut my mouth and keep quiet. It hurt to grow up in my home.

One weekend I parked my convertible on Santa Monica Boulevard. There were crowds of teenagers walking the street and driving their cars. A young brunette stopped next to my car. She climbed into the driver's side of my convertible and seated herself on my lap. "Let's talk about the first thing that pops up," she said. Even in that optimal situation, and experiencing penile lust, I was reluctant to respond appropriately.

I went to California in 1966. Before I departed and returned home, I'd copulated with a dozen females, but I asked none of them for a date. Vaguely I remember penile lust induced by female images within my own mind, but not by those actual coital partners. I didn't form an attachment with any of those girls.

During my sojourn in California, I often phoned my lover, Sharon. A memory-image of Sharon's vaginal fluids inhabited my mind and brain. As I returned home, there were few of the miles between California and Maryland when I wasn't imaging Sharon accompanied by genital swelling.

After arriving in Maryland, I attempted to rebuild my life. This time, I worked in a men's wear store. Although I spoke with Sharon, our pairbond would never be the same. Nonetheless, it required another ten years for the mental images of her to fade.

Females were as erotically inclined toward me as I was toward them, yet I still found myself watching stripteasers and spending money on prostitutes. I'd take my weekly earnings and visit Baltimore's Block. Watching was all I could do.

The men's wear store at which I worked was located in a mall in Towson, Maryland. Girls were available. I dated many of them. I also had one experience most men can only wish they had. One evening after leaving work I stopped to get a drink. Besides the bartender there was only one other person at the bar, an attractive lady who appeared much older than myself.

She introduced herself as Stacy. She bought me a drink. Then she asked me to go home with her for fifty dollars. I accepted her lustful invitation, but only because I was already horny. At that time of my life, I didn't know anything about sexology, so I didn't know that I could fall in love only with women who were much younger than myself. However, that didn't matter, for salacious images of several girls I had observed that day were already spurring my penile lust.

Coital activity with Stacy was orgasmic but not euphoric. I received a request to return for a repeat episode, but I never did. After all, although I did not know it yet, my genital response concerning money was a secondary paraphilia, not a primary one. If my genital arousal were voluntary, I could have made a fortune with older women. Furthermore, if I were a gerontophile, genitally aroused by older women, instead of an ephebophile, genitally aroused by younger women, I'd be a gigolo.

During the Christmas season, the men's wear store was busy. I enjoyed those days and nights, for there was no time to indulge in paraphilic imagery. Then I encountered an adorable girl: Keri. She had her Christmas list and sought my help in selecting gifts for those on her list. After the store closed, I met Keri for a drink. Both of us were horny. Consequently, we became coital partners. Our partnership was not incited by reciprocal love, however. I think that neither one of us knew anything about the state of love.

Subsequently, our coital insouicience led to Keri's pregnancy. She didn't want or need a baby, nor did I, although our reasons for seeking an abortion were different. I didn't want to subject a child to this foul world. Keri had already had two children whom she had surrendered for adoption. We arranged for the abortion, which cost me two hundred dollars. That's at least one child who won't be born into this hell which we call earth.

Our distorted attachment waned after Keri's abortion. I got a second job and moved to Brooklyn Park, Maryland. Then my paraphilia of masochism began dictating my behavior again. I felt an irrepressible urge to spank myself in accord with the imagery of my vandalized lovemap. Again without my consent, on occasions while working at the clothing store, I'd be imaging spanking scenes. My genitalia would swell and ooze genital fluid. Throughout the day my masochistic lust would dispose me to enacting the spanking scenario upon my arrival home. My masochistic ideation would locate the proper instrument to spank myself with, the proper position to perform the ritual in, and the appropriate mental scenes to image. With hindsight, I'm amazed at how specific the scenario needed to be for optimal orgasm.

I couldn't lash or paddle my buttocks harshly enough. There was always a frustrated feeling because my arm tired while spanking myself. Also, I longed to hear a cruel voice demand that I hold my buttocks still while being punished. I had a relentless urging to find a dominatrix for a better spanking. I also always had a dread of exposure.

At times, I had strength to resist the paraphilic intrusion. I'd repeat the word, no, over and over again. But no amount of opposition worked. My paraphilia rebelled with an immobilizing effect. I wouldn't be able to walk. Eventually, it stopped me from performing any activity until I surrendered. Then, after my masochized orgasm, I'd wonder why I had resisted. My orgasm always seemed worth dying for.

At twenty-four years of age, I contemplated marriage to a girl named Karen. She was a recent college graduate. On our third date, Karen asked if I liked her, for I hadn't tried to kiss her. At that time, I didn't know why I was disinclined to kiss her. I explained my behavior as respect for her as a person, and not as a sex object. In fact, Karen didn't spur me to lust, and I enjoyed that. Genital arousal didn't make me happy.

After six months of dating, Karen and I married. Our coital activity was frequent, but my coital lust wasn't in response to Karen's morphology or physique. My penile lust was faciltated by the female images I observed throughout my day at work. That vicarious arousal facilitated the distorted concept of being in love, whereas neither of us knew anything about that state. Like everyone else we thought that being in love meant an active desire for someone. Fortunately, today I know better.

The worst event of our marriage soon occurred: pregnancy. I didn't want any children, but she wanted to give her parents a grandchild. If I were to accept a baby, it would have to be a female. When the baby arrived, it was a boy.

Facing my responsibility, I strived to be a good father and husband. Ater all, I wanted to make my son's life better than my own. Unfortunately, I was unaware of how my bipolar disorder would ruin my best intentions.

As parents with a child, we required a babysitter. That was not a problem, for our neighborhood was occupied by families with many young girls. Most of them were precocious teenagers. My life would have been better had I known of ephebophilia, with its characteristic fixation on young women. Our first babysitter was a nubile brunette, fifteen years of age. I was not a "dirty old man," nor was I a pervert. Yet, in the proximity of our babysitter, Laura, my genitals swelled instantly. Then, like an intrusive invader, her form and image centered itself on my mental stage. Suddenly, and irrespective of my marital state, I longed to speak with her. I was eager to charm her. My mind's imaging posed her as receptive to my lustiness. I didn't willfully desire a partnership of love and lust with her. The desire occurred without my consent. I might have been orgasmic with her, but never happy.

Laura's teenaged body was ideally pretty. She flirted with me in my wife's absence. When she pushed her firm breasts against my chest, my penile fluid oozed onto the inside of my trousers. I felt an intense ambivalence. Although I yearned to release my erect penis and copulate with her, somehow I resisted. Today, in hindsight, I know that she was only a partial parallel to my ephebophilic lovemap. Optimal arousal genitally occurs only with women between the ages of seventeen and twenty-seven.

One day I was home alone. I was seated in an armchair facing my couch. Then, without any effort on my part, I was picturing Laura kneeling on the couch with her buttocks naked and red from a spanking. That projected image of Laura swelled my penis instantly. I masturbated for an hour with similar imagery inhabiting my mental stage. The orgasm was overwhelming. Subsequently, I knew that I ought to find an escape from ephebophilic lust before it ruined me.

Trying to escape, I sought a paramour. I searched the clubs of Baltimore's Block. Eventually I picked up the girl named Nora. She was a hooker who liked me and needed my money. Moreover, her facial features, physique, and youthfulness spurred me to optimal lustfulness. I made arrangements to copulate with her once a week. Our copulation was oral, vaginal, and anal. Furthermore, our lustbond was reciprocal. As a result, I experienced over twenty orgasms per week, some with my wife and some with Nora.

Even after a year, Karen didn't suspect my lust affair with Nora. I overheard Karen tell a friend over the telephone that we had a great sex life. Karen assumed that because of our frequent coitus my sex life was great. The truth was that my coital activity with Karen was incited by my imagery of Nora. My affectional love was with Karen, and my genital lust was with Nora. Moreover, I could spank Nora, but I couldn't spank Karen. Today, in hindsight, I know that my love and lust were split.

After four years of marriage, I owned a house, two cars, and used twenty credit cards. My son was healthy and growing fast. We fit the appearance of an ideal American family, but it was appearance only, and paraphilically doomed. Meantime, I frequently wondered how a man could abandon his home, wife, and family for another woman. Then it happened. Over nothing more than orgasmic lust, I was doomed to sacrifice everything.

On a snowy December night, Nora and I abandoned our families. My paraphilic lust deceived me into thinking that Nora and I were in the state of love. With the knowledge of hindsight, I know that I was in a paraphilic fugue state. Perhaps Nora was too. We traveled three hundred miles before we stopped for the night. During the drive, Nora's hand played with my penis with few interruptions. My psychophysical energy couldn't be abated.

We spent about six hours swiving and quimming, taking turns at working out, and being worked upon. Even before I studied sexology, I felt uncomfortable labeling coital activity as making love. After all, love doesn't cause genital arousal, but lust does. In the case of our coital partnership, genital lust overpowered affectional love.

The more I spanked Nora, the more she yearned to quim my penis. I'd chain her to a bed with her thighs spread widely, then I'd swive her until my penis and my whole body collapsed. Our paraphilic lust-bond evaporated all concern for abandoned homes and families.

With Nora, my paraphilic fugue states recurred constantly for about two years. There was no counting the frequency with which our genital arousal was activated. Our longing, eagerness, and inclination was for fellatio, cunnilingus, and genital fondling, as well as penis-in-vagina action. Our talk was eroticized. Our rituals were of paraphilic spanking. We were indifferent to actuality outside of our lustbond.

As our paraphilic lust eventually waned, there was an insufficient residual lovebond to sustain our partnership. Nora concerned herself again with her son whom she had abandoned. My sense of economic accountability reestablished itself. Both Nora and I experienced mental imagery of other partners who aroused us genitally. Then came the day when we didn't spur each other to lust at all. A confused partnership is all that remained.

Nora returned to Baltimore without me. Shortly thereafter, I too returned to Baltimore. Three years earlier we couldn't survive one hour without touching or talking to each other. In Baltimore, we established a companionate partnership. Nora did not appear on my mental screen as an incitement to lust ever again.

I was introduced to three of Nora's sisters. My lustfulness was aroused by two of them, and we shared genital sex. The third sister's age and physique matched my lovemap, but her demeanor was contrary to it. It was an unrequited love, and alas one I'll always regret.

I was back where I had started. I kept going through economic, romantic, and inexplicable moody phases. Psychologist and psychiatrist couldn't help me. I visited several without favorable results. I know now that I needed a sexologist.

I began another business. My ability to sell a tangible product in unchartered territory was unparalleled. At the outset, my somewhat manic energy level eliminated prolonged rest. Then, as if possessed, I felt an urging to spend money on women, especially stripteasers and hookers. I worked all day and spent the nights watching stripteasers.

I encountered the same old criticism. I yearned to gaze or stare at the naked female. Hookers assume that all men want to copulate with them. If a man wants anything beside an orgasm within a vagina, he's viewed as perverted, such are the distorted and exaggerated concepts of maleness. To be labeled perverted for enjoying a woman without touching her—who wants that?

Since I was spending great sums of money, I needed to sustain my earnings. After a year of selling, I covered four different states with my product. One night I stayed at a motel out of town. When my eyes opened in the morning, I couldn't move. At first I assumed that I was dreaming and closed my eyes. But when I opened my eyes again, I remained immobile.

Eventually, and with a mountain of effort, I reached the telephone, which was only one foot away on the night table. I phoned a local hospital and arranged for an emergency evaluation. In the hospital, I was given a series of tests and a thorough workup. The diagnosis was rendered. I had the bipolar disorder, otherwise known as being manic-depressive.

This diagnosis explained much of the history of my behavior. It explained why, on some days, I experienced limited psychophysical energy. Then, on other days, I was disinclined to perform any task. Erroneously, I had attributed my low energy to a vitamin deficiency. My mother had done the same thing. Now I realized that my coital and orgasmic activity were episodes in synchrony with bipolar disorder. I realized also that my suicidal attitudes and behavior were likewise attributable to bipolar disorder.

Upon discharge from the hospital, I was taking the medication lithium carbonate. Truly I felt much better. Inadequately informed about my newly discovered disorder, I finished the bottle of lithium, and then ceased its usage. That was a mistake that I'd live to regret. I did not know of the genetic origin of, or predisposition toward, bipolar disorder, nor that it will always be with me in some way, manner, or degree.

Without lithium, I drifted back to my way of living from one orgasm to the next. How can I explain it, except that it felt good? So how could anything be wrong? My multiple orgasms weren't, however, my only source of feeling wonderful or euphoric. When the manic phase of my bipolar disorder was uppermost, it produced a high that was very high. Of course, the problem was my inability to turn the phases on or off.

Perhaps the most perplexing behavior of my life was spending my money on women, even when there were women available to reciprocate in coital activity for free. There were many times when I found that if I couldn't pay for sexualized activity, I couldn't enjoy it. I even imposed a payment situation on women with whom it was totally unnecessary.

I've escaped the hell into which I was born, but I'll always carry the scars from it. Currently, I'm the survivor of an error in my genetic code, a vandalized lovemap, social miscasting, a misguided trial, and a senseless prison term. Through an onerous struggle, I've deprived those childhood vandals of a final victory in my life. I'm in charge now. Regrettably, however, I'm a lifetime paraphile, and I must carry it to my grave, always vigilant for the signs of an incipient relapse.

6

Incarcerated Orgasms
Prison Research

During seven years of my incarceration, I have counted over two thousand orgasms. In prison that's what inmates do. They fuck in their brains. The motion between the hand and the penis is merely a manifestation of that which is being staged in their mental theaters. They're rehearsing! Their orgasms are the climaxes to their X-rated mental videos. Their mental scenarios are the collective imagery of the past and the prelude to future scenes of lustfulness.

If an inmate's impetus to lust is dominating his female partner, he'll rehearse that to perfection on his mind's stage. If an inmate's lust is spurred by raping and murdering little boys, prison will allow him to refine that paraphilic expression. If the inmate's rehearsal pictures are of his watching his wife being copulated by other men, then that's what he'll practice again when he is released. But he'll have the advantage of leisurely rehearsal of his incarcerated orgasms.

I recall Marvin, an ethnic inmate who raped a nonethnic female. He was incarcerated. During his three years of incarcerated orgasms, he raped his victim on his mental stage. When the parole board released him, he traveled over two states and raped the same woman. He could have raped a dozen other women. But his particular paraphilia, stigmatophilia, predisposed him to return and rape the woman with whom he had rehearsed the rape in his incarcerated orgasms.

Sidney didn't socialize with many of the inmates during our time in the recreation hall, although that changed when movies of war, destruction, and explosives appeared on television. Then he couldn't restrain himself from talking. I didn't know what his conviction was, but I sensed that he was a paraphile.

Most inmates will talk freely about those things with which they feel comfortable, so I sought an opportunity to examine the contents of his lovemap by questioning him. It worked. When I asked him how to make a bomb, he couldn't stop talking. Here was a man who wanted to reveal something, and I was there to listen.

I asked Sidney what he had been convicted for. He grinned. Then, he said, "That bitch, I got her good."

"What did she do?" I inquired, "And to whom are you referring?"

"My dead girlfriend," he said, then paused. "That bomb I told you about, well I put it in her kitchen. It reacts to heat, like the heat in her oven. She didn't want to see me anymore. But I couldn't stop imagining scenes of her. I kept thinking of her with another guy. I wanted to get both of them."

In an effort to keep him talking, I said, "Maybe she was not in love with you anymore. Love does perish, you know."

"She told me she'd always love me," Sidney snarled, "I couldn't stop thinking about her, especially her and that guy. While I walked around with a hard-on, he was fucking her. So I broke into her house.

"I put the heat-sensitive bomb into the bottom of her oven. Later, that night, I parked down the street. I saw her new boyfriend go into her place. There I was, holding my dick while he's getting some pussy, I stopped that. About an hour after he went into her house, the kitchen was blown to bits."

Sidney smiled.

"How did the police connect you with the bomb?" I asked.

"Oh, somebody saw my car parked on the street. They reported it, saying a man was masturbating in his car," Sidney replied in disgust.

"Were you jerking off?" I asked.

"I just couldn't stop seeing her with that guy in my mind," retorted Sidney. "Nobody will fuck her now."

In fact, Sidney ceased imagining his former girfriend right after she died. Sidney was spurred to lust by stage managing a disaster. It was directly connected to his orgasm. He's a symphorophile. Of course, no one made the connection between Sidney's genital lust and the bombing of his estranged girlfriend's house.

I noticed Sal because he was always selling something. He'd steal something from one inmate, then sell it, or barter it with another inmate. Compulsive behavior fascinated me, for the compulsive person couldn't help it. And I had to know why.

I had bartered a few things with Sal so I approached him in the prison yard. He spoke spontaneously. I asked him what he did to be in prison. He was convicted of burglary. Somehow I knew that was only an ostensible charge.

"You want to know how I got caught?" asked Sal, as though he wanted to talk about it. "This is going to sound weird, but don't laugh at me, will you? I saw a girl walking along a street. I watched to see which house she'd enter. For a couple of days I drove by the house. She was real young, but she gave me a real hard-on. Anyhow, when I drove by this one time, there weren't any cars parked outside. So I broke in through the basement window. Coming through the door onto the first floor, I saw the girl sleeping on the couch. First I looked around for something to steal, but I couldn't keep my mind off the sleeping girl.

"I crawled next to the couch where she slept. Sneaking my hand under her slip, I rubbed the outside of her panties. I had one hell of a hard-on. Then, just when I got off, she woke up. She got a real good look at me. By the time I got up, she was banging on the next door neighbor's house. You know how it is after you have an orgasm, it takes a couple of minutes to revive yourself.

"Well, by the time I got to my car and started down the street, the cops were everywhere. They charged me with attempted rape and burglary. I beat the rape charge, but got stuck with the burglary charge," Sal concluded, with a sigh.

Fortunately, I'd just been reading about somnophilia. This is the sleeping princess syndrome. Sal's lust was activated by fondling the genitalia of a sleeping girl, either in imagery or actuality.

Sal's story started in early childhood. "When I was three years of age my mother would call me into her bedroom," Sal said. "She'd tell me to put my hand between her thighs. Then she ordered me to insert my fingers into her vagina. She moved around a lot, but wouldn't let me move my fingers. Finally, when she stopped squirming on the bed, she'd slap me for having my hand between her thighs. But she made me do it until I was ten years old. I was damned if I did and damned if I didn't."

I met an inmate named Bernard at the Maryland Correctional Institution in Hagerstown. I had just arrived and was visiting the rec hall for the first time. When I stepped into the large room, someone spoke to me as though he knew me. The inmate insisted that he knew me from the Maryland State Penitentiary, but I'd never been confined there. Bernard couldn't keep his eyes off my crotch.

I challanged him to a game of chess. I rarely lose, but I let Bernard win to discover his conviction and his obvious paraphilia. Bernard had been charged with forty-four counts of rape. He was convicted of only a dozen of them. This was his forth term in prison since the onset of puberty. He was just as comfortable in prison as he was outside of it. He was bisexual, but with an interesting twist. The heterosexual side of his paraphilic lust raped women older than himself. His intermale lust raped men younger than himself. Whether his distorted lust was genitogenital or anogenital, it had to be coercive. Literally, the terror in the older women or younger men was for him the impetus to genital arousal. Bernard's paraphilia was threefold. A fixation for older women, a fixation for younger men, and copulation that had to be forced, not reciprocal. Bernard longed for my asshole, but since he couldn't menace or frighten me, he stopped pursuing me as a lustmate.

Mitchell was tall, lean, bearded, and quiet. We were playing chess. I had won four games in a row. "What did they get you for?" I asked.

"Some old lady said that I raped her," he replied, while trying to get out of check.

"Do you mean old lady as in older than yourself?" I inquired. Then he got out of check.

"Yeah, she was seventy-six years old," he said, then smiled because he had gotten out of check.

"Was it a bum rap, or are you guilty?" I questioned, while he protected his king with his bishop.

"I did it, but I don't remember all of it. I was drunk," he said, with a disgusted look on his face.

Evidentally, Mitchell had been overcome by his fixation on older women: gerontophilia. He drank to cope with his paraphilic lust. He was only twenty-five years of age. He couldn't understand why he had a hard-on for a seventy-six-year-old woman. The court never concerned itself about his odd fixation on an older woman. It just sentenced him without any thought to his sexual disorder as paraphile with geronto-philia. Mitchell's act of rape had nothing to do with power or control over the older woman. His vandalized lovemap predisposed him to the aged, without his own consent or fulfillment.

I was moved into the cell next to Shad. He called out of his cell window to me. He wanted to look at my lust magazines. That's what he called erotica. I was not inclined to loan my magazines to inmates, especially since they will cut pictures out of them. They'll claim that they were that way when they received them.

To gain my trust he sent me one of his own erotic magazines. When I sent the magazine back, he tried to use his trust of me to get one of my magazines. But I wasn't going to be deceived. He took umbrage at my distrust and called to the inmate in the cell above mine, instructing him to pour water down the wall so it would enter my cell. Contrary to his interpretation of my demeanor, I become defiant when intimidated, not timid. When he discovered that I wouldn't surrender my magazines, he gave up.

On another day I overheard him recalling for another inmate the circumstances of his arrest. He stalked a girl who lived alone. There he assaulted her brutally and genitally. "I made her bend over while I fucked her asshole," he boasted. "She didn't like that a bit, but I sure did." Before he departed, he threatened her with death if she reported him to the police. His intimidation was successful.

Shad returned to rape her repeatedly. Of course, there was deficient genital lust unless he forced her into what he considered degrading sexual behavior. "I made that bitch suck my dick while I watched her television, and ate her food," he disclosed, with cruel delight.

Finally, after seven other episodes of his biastophilic rape in the same neighborhood, a victim called the police. Basically, rape is coital coercion, but Shad as a biastophilic rapist had to have a humiliated and terrified victim. His genital arousal was dependent upon mental scenes or actual scenes of dominating and copulating with struggling victims, especially those who are beaten or threatened into capitulation. These scenarios were the eliciting stimulus to his distorted lustfulness. He is serving fifty years for rape. However, prison won't alter his bia-stophilic fantasy sex. In fact, prison is perfect as a fertile ground for the mental rehearsal of future episodes of rape.

Stu was a predator of the human being. In outside society men who are troublemakers or predators can be avoided—sometimes. In prison you're stuck with them. Stu didn't concern himself with the sex of the individuals he attacked. He was in prison for robbery, rape, and assault. He's a paraphile, and the state paroled him. Before he left, he told the story of one of his charges.

"One night, I forced my way into a house. This old man and woman tried to hold their back door shut as I forced it open. I beat the hell out of the old man once I got the door open. They had a granddaughter visiting them, so after I tied up her grandparents, I took her into the bedroom and raped her. She was a virgin. I fucked her so hard that the sheet was soaked with blood.

"I packed up things of the grandparents to sell. Then, just before I left, I fucked that little bitch again. I had to beat the hell out of her to keep her quiet. Then,I took their car keys, loaded their car, and split. I figured the little bitch could untie her grandparents."

I figured that he is a marauding and predatory paraphile. He raped the girl because he was spurred to lust by stealing. So he's a klepto-phile, too. His vandalized lovemap requires him to break into a residence and steal from strangers. While stealing property, he may also steal the usage of a female victim's vagina. Nonetheless, his incitement to lustfulness is stealing, not raping.

Les was quite gregarious. He knew that I studied sexology. He also knew that his behavioral sex wasn't typical. One day, he asked me if I liked an officer who was a petite female. I said that I had no inclination for her erotically. Les responded: "Every time I jerk off, I imagine myself sticking my dick up her asshole. It ain't fun for me unless she don't like getting a dick up her ass."

I asked Les about his experiences before his incarceration. I wanted to know the connections between now and then. "In high school, I knew this girl who liked me," he said. "The only time I felt good about her is when I pushed her away or told her she ain't worth a fuck.

"When I got a girl into debt, I'd threaten her with great physical harm or she'd have to let me fuck her. I enjoyed humiliating her, and keeping her my private sex slave. If they like what I'm doing to them my dick gets soft."

All indications are that Les is a paraphilic sadist, a biastophile. His lust, which is manifested as genital arousal, is maximized by domination and humiliation of the partner. As I listened to his experiences, and the imagery of his incarcerated orgasms, it was clear. Les had to be the authority who imposed abuse, torture, punishment, discipline, humiliation, obedience, and servitude upon others, especially women.

Jerry showed me two pictures of his girlfriend while we were waiting in line at the institutional commissary. According to his ideal, she was quite attractive. Jerry's own facial features and physique were also quite ideal. I'm the first person to admit that looks can be deceiving, so I longed to know the circumstances of his arrest and conviction. "With an adorable girlfriend like that, what are you doing in prison?" I asked, with a puzzled look on my face.

"My mother asked the same question," Jerry replied, repeating his mother's question: "Why did you rape a girl when you've got your own pretty girlfriend?"

"One night, this buddy of mine and I picked up a girl. The three of us were talking and joking while he drove. He stopped the car near a wooded area. My buddy started to kiss the girl and feel her up. She resisted. He told me to hold her arms. While I held her arms, my buddy tore her clothes off and slapped her face. The funny thing is that I didn't get a hard-on until we forced her into fucking. After my buddy dragged her out of the car and raped her, I raped her. She kept screaming so we beat her to shut her up. Then, while we were having a few beers, she ran toward the road. A car stopped and picked her up. Later we were arrested. But I don't know why I raped her."

Afterward, I observed an inmate exiting the commissary with a large bag of purchased items. The inmate was well known as a homosexual. Stopping where Jerry stood, he said, "I got everything you asked for." That's when I discovered Jerry's bisexuality.

It took me several more months before I guessed at his ratio of love and lust with the female, and his ratio of love and lust with the male. It appeared that his heterosexual lust was dominant with his girlfriend and other women. But homosexual love dominated him with men.

When I asked Jerry about his intergenital activities with his girlfriend, he said, "She liked me and my mother liked her. She was available when I had a hard-on so I fucked her. But I don't think that I was in love with her."

Since the gauge for love's state is that one's partner be pictured on one's mental stage as an impetus to both lust and love, Jerry didn't qualify for being in love. He never imagined his girlfriend and himself in coital activity. In fact, he reported that during their intergenital sex, their lubrication failed. It wasn't until mental images of forcing a female to fuck appeared on his mental stage that his penile fluid flowed, thereby facilitating their sexual activity.

His intermale love was manifested in prison. With or without genital lust, he'd let male partners penetrate his anal cavity. Jerry is a paraphile. He needs help, not incarceration.

Dan spoke lustfully of women. He was quite extroverted. But fucking women wasn't his primary impetus to lustfulness. I told him about my tendency toward a hairless pudenda during cunnilingus. He sought the taste of a hairy cunt for cunnilingus, especially one permeated with bodily odor. "When my girlfriend takes a shit, I follow her into the bathroom," he disclosed. "While she sits on the toilet shitting, I lick her cunt. When she's finished, I clean her anus with my tongue. Eating her shit turns me on," Dan said, as his face glowed from coprophilic memory.

At that time, there was a transvestite on the tier, Robyn. Dan was pairbonded with Robyn. He didn't have a fixation for men in women's clothing. He paired with Robyn for anal copulation. "The fact that Robyn is really a man doesn't bother me, because Robyn looks and acts like a woman," he said. "I hang out with Robyn so I can dig in her ass." Robyn's paraphilia was transacting orgasms for money, or in this case commissary items. Most inmates viewed Robyn as homosexual, but behavioral sex with men was not Robyn's impetus to lust. Dan coaxed Robyn with gifts and treated the transvestite like the woman that Robyn appeared to be. Receiving gifts was part of being loved by a man as far as Robyn was concerned. Alas, they both died of AIDS.

The Division of Corrections causes great disorientation in inmates by moving them from one cell to another, or from one institution to another. The following incident was blown out of proportion because of the unknown.

I was unfamiliar with most of the inmates on the tier. Standing near my cell door, I waited for the door to be unlocked from the lockbox at the end of the tier. Inmates were bantering as they usually do. Suddenly, I felt a hand grasp at my crotch. When I turned to detect the guilty person, he ran away, striving to avoid detection. It was Tod.

After three years of experience within the walls of prison, I was cautious. If I didn't report the inmate's grasping of my crotch, he'd assume that I was in favor of it, and do it again. If I retaliated by fighting him, to indicate my disapproval of his playing with me, I'd end up with an assault charge. By reflection, I made my decision to report the incident to an institutional officer. Of course, by reporting anything to the officer in charge, I'd be labeled a coward and snitch. I was damned if I did, and damned if I didn't. Being discrete in prison is an indication of weakness, even to the officers.

After my reporting Tod's targeted touching of my groin, a hearing was scheduled within the next ninety-six hours. During those hours I discovered Tod's paraphilia and bieroticism. Disclosing the events that led to his incarceration, Tod said, "I didn't rape anybody as the police charged me with. I felt this crazy urge to pat the bottoms of the women in the Giant food store. So I ran through the store rubbing the skirts of five or six female shoppers. I got more attention than I expected. People were running after me, so I found a house to hide in. When I broke into the house, an old lady was there. I struggled with her. I had a hard-on from those women in the store. Momentarily I thought about sticking my dick into the old lady to get off. But after she screamed, I lost my erection. When I attempted to hide someplace else, I got caught. The old lady said that I tried to rape her."

"So why did you grasp me in the crotch?" I inquired.

"I thought that you wouldn't mind. Somehow you turned me on like those women in the grocery store did," said Tod. This was not the first time he had grasped the crotch of an inmate. The prison had charged him with sexual assault on two previous occasions. At the hearing, I asked to have my charge dismissed. I attempted to explain Tod's paraphilia of toucheurism to the hearing officer, but it didn't work. As a result, Tod was convicted with sexual assault, and for the third time. Considering his twenty years for attempted rape and his sexual assault charges in prison, Tod may serve most of his sentence. However, he is not an assaultive inmate, not a rapist. That's clearly indicated by his failed erection after breaking into the old lady's house. If he were a rapist, the woman's terror would have incited rape, not discouraged it. Tod's paraphilia is fulfilled only by the surreptitious touching of a partner's erotic parts. He was not dangerous. He could have been treated without the cost of incarcerations. But Tod did not know about treatment. He did not even know that he had a sexological disorder that had a name. The existence and name of his disorder was also unknown to the correctional authorities. Like hundreds of other prisoners, Tod was in prison for the wrong reason, charged with an offense that masks an underlying paraphilic sexological disorder that is never brought to the surface in court.

I was on segregation. It was filthy there. Supposedly, there weren't any other cells available. Only two inmates were allowed out of their cells and onto the tier at the same time. I met an inmate, Harry. He was in his fifties. He asked me what I did to occupy my time on that dreadful tier.

"I study paraphilic sexology," I said, and explained what it is. We walked around rat defecation. That was difficult for Harry, he walked with a crutch. At the far end of the tier, we paused.

"Do you know why I'm in here?" Harry asked.

"I know that it pertains to paraphilic sexology," I replied, with a look that allowed him to rest with his guilt.

"I raped a little girl, and she died, but I didn't mean for her to die," said Harry, as a tear rolled down his face. Obviously, he was a pedophile. I asked Harry how the little girl died.

"Well, I didn't mean to rape her. She was a neighbor girl. I was in my garage. She walked into the garage and asked my name. I started talking to her. We were alone. I had this terrible urge to undress her. I had a hard-on. I don't know why, but I asked her if she'd ever seen a man's dick. She didn't know what I was talking about. When I unzipped my pants to show it to her, she screamed. I panicked. I grabbed her to stop her from screaming. When I saw her panties, I couldn't stop myself from pulling them off. I yelled at her to shut up. I hit her, and she stopped screaming, I figured she was unconscious and wouldn't know if I fucked her. I can't believe that I fucked her. I hadn't had an erection in months. I was taking medication for my leg, and I couldn't get it up. When I tried to revive her, I then realized that I'd killed her. I called the police and turned myself in. They called me a pervert."

I instructed Harry to contact the Sexual Disorders Clinic at The Johns Hopkins Hospital. He seemed grateful for that information. Our walk was over so we returned to our cells.

Early in the morning I heard loud voices. By sticking my mirror out of my cell, I caught the activities at the end of the tier in my mirror. Somebody said, "He's dead." Harry had choked himself on the end of his crutch. Literally, he had rammed the narrow end of his crutch down his throat. He had died over a paraphilic orgasm. He didn't intend for that little girl to die, but paraphilias don't give a damn!

Epilogue
Output of Discovery

I've put my enforced leisure to good use. It facilitated my unexpected discoveries. I felt an urgency. I was determined to benefit from every day of introspection. Mostly, I intended to discover the states of love. I was enraged over my ignorance. "What is this damn thing called love?" I asked myself. The way people bandy about the word *love,* you'd conclude that it was the most ill-defined concept on earth.

The police drew a composite sketch of me prior to my arrest. I was amazed at how accurate it was. It occurred to me that lovemaps are just that: composite images. My prepubertal brain devised composite images of those partners with whom I'd fall in love. Postpubertally, I did fall in love. But my lovemap, with its composite imagery, had been vandalized. I didn't know that. Thus, my state of love was always altered or distorted. Unknowingly, my lust wasn't modified by affectionate love. That's the role of love, to modify genital lust.

As I have already related, the partnership between my playmate and me was severed. That misguided severing indefinitely halted my pairing, partnering, or pairbonding with any female partner. My affectionate attachment to future lovers went into hibernation. But my developing lustfulness continued to develop, void of that affectionate love. That day and hour marked the outset of the vandalizing of my lovemap. It took another forty years for the pairbonding of love to emerge from hibernation.

Although not everything is known about visual imprinting in the infant, I suppose that it commences the minute the infant's eyes open. My imprinted images predisposed me to the state of love after the onset of puberty, but love did not materialize. That's why many of the partners with whom I thought I'd fallen in love were partners I didn't really like. That's an impairment of love's state.

Before being estranged from my playmate, Pam, I experienced an imprint. That imprint was my sister's vulva. Unfortunately, it wasn't connected with the full range of heterosexual partnering. The imprinted vulva was out of place in time. Today, I'm genitally aroused by the sight of a hairless vulva. When the interconnection is made between my imprinted vulva, and a girl's actual vulva, my penis swells. It's spontaneous, and isn't connected to a specific female.

The cleavage of my affectionate love from genital lust was set before I had viewed even one piece of commercial erotica. This cleavage happened inadvertently, for even these forty years later no one in my entire family knows what the state of love is. So they couldn't have vandalized my lovemap deliberately. If they had known about lovemaps and vandalized lovemaps, I probably wouldn't have ended up with my former dominatrix.

Conceivably, my imprinting could have disposed me to paraphilic murder, rape, stealing, elaborate deception, arson, amputation, sadism, self-murder, self-strangulation, impersonating a baby, eating shit, fondling buttocks, copulating with animals, and so on. Instead, I became imprinted to masochism.

Watching my imaginal scenarios was frequently confusing. I didn't dismiss any scenario as insignificant. After all, I didn't put the images in my head. I didn't form, arrange, or reconstruct them. I merely watched my mind's theater and took notes. Eventually, I discovered a parallel in Betty, from my seventh grade class. She was the first classmate whose lustful assertiveness toward me proved that I was attractive to women. She probably knew why she was horny for me, but I didn't.

I wrote the story about Betty several times before it made the final draft of this book. I sought to know the interconnection between my imprinting and Betty. If my penile arousal occurs in proximity of a girl, it's because of lovemap imprinting. I longed to discover why I responded to her, especially since she didn't resemble my mother or sisters. I'd be in bad shape if my penis swelled in relation to all women.

Suddenly it happened. Like a subliminal advertisement on a movie screen, I recognized a face in relation to Betty. It was the face of a lady in my childhood neighborhood. I'd forgotten about her because she had died. But that's the mystery of imprinting. You never know when it happens, and it's not a lovemap imprint unless it induces genital arousal.

There was nothing wrong with that lady's imprinted face. But my pairbonding had been impaired after Pam, and before Betty. So when I encountered Betty's actual image, my penis perked immediately. An interconnection had been made. I should have fallen in love with Betty, and if I had we would have been boyfriend and girlfriend.

Betty's image interchanged with my lovemap imprint. That incited my penile arousal. But my affectionate love was still in abeyance. Therefore, I couldn't reciprocate Betty's eagerness to unite our love and lust in an erotic partnership. My love and lust didn't coexist. As I now recall Betty, she was ideally sensual, adorable, delicious, delectable, and erotic. If I could live that event over, I'd bury my penile erection in Betty's vagina. And that's what she longed for, then. I wasn't stupid or unattractive, but my lovemap was vandalized. It controlled me, I didn't control it.

Object imprinting starts before one's language defines an interrelationship. Perhaps if I'd been taught about pairbonded love and lust I might have coped with my situation better than I did. A language of eroticism and erotic partnerships might have allowed me to copulate with Betty, but avoid pregnancy. Rehearsal with Betty might have brought my hibernating affectionate love out of hibernation before it was too late.

Meanwhile, as I tuned in to my imaginal scenarios, I noticed a shunting of scenes. For example, I'd be with a girl in an erotic scene. My phallus would be erecting. But in order for my lustfulness to maximize, my mental scenery shunted to a scene of spankings. My penile lust didn't function with affectionate love. I discovered that by examining my own imagery or mental pictures.

I was reluctant to use the word fantasy in my research, especially without qualifying it appropriately. It implies something unreal. I noticed it in books, magazines, and on television as though it has no basis in fact. Or it was suggestive of something sexual as though there is something wrong with being a sex, or one of the sexes.

After six consecutive years of introspective self-observation, I've discovered the scenes, scenarios, images, characters, and words within my mind to be real. Nonetheless, there is a vast difference between an erotic fantasy and a nonerotic fantasy. The erotic or eroticized fantasy possesses great significance. It can forecast your heterosexual, bisexual, or homosexual behavior. Moreover, a paraphilic fantasy is downright precise. And I have no idea what a sexual fantasy is, except that I'm a sex having a fantasy, perhaps. A nonerotic fantasy won't induce genital swelling, but an erotic fantasy will. A nonerotic fantasy can be trivial or exaggerated, but without affectionate love or genital arousal.

With the knowledge that my love is split from my lust, I used the terms *pairbonded love* or *pairbonded lust*. A fantasy or imaginal scenario of pairbonded love failed to induce genital arousal. So it could be misconstrued as a nonerotic fantasy. However, a pairbonded love fantasy would invariably depict or picture lovers, pairs, couples, or partners doing what lovers do, but without manifestations of lustfulness.

I found it impossible to continue my research without using the verb *to pairbond* or its variants: *a pairbond, pairbonded, pairbonding,* or *pairbondedness*. These are much better than a word like *relationship,* which could refer to a relationship with anything. *Partnership* is a good replacement for relationship. A pairbond refers to partners, couples, mates, lovers, and married or nonmarried people. After all, that's what life is all about, the pairing, partnering, or pairbonding of human beings. Furthermore, the pairbond between a mother and infant is the prelude to the pairbondage of girlfriend and boyfriend, lover and lover, or husband and wife. Moreover, pairbonding is part of the brain's pathways. It is predisposed in the human being.

At first, I found the examination of my paraphilic fantasies discouraging. My penis wouldn't swell, nor could I achieve an orgasm without mental scenes of ephebophilic girls being spanked. In some scenarios, I was being spanked by a dominatrix. But there was the possibility that I might discover something new about the paraphilias, so I continued my research into my own paraphilia. Alas, I also realized that millions of women suffer because of men who are paraphiles. Frequently I was thankful that I was not a paraphilic rapist (colloquially known as a serial rapist), murderer (colloquially known as a serial killer), and so on. Although it wasn't much of an option or alternative, my paraphilic lust was based on subjective or objective spanking, mostly.

One day, in an intuitional moment of enlightenment, this question impinged upon my mind: "Could I viably and properly conclude that affectionate love, in whatever ratio, is the modifier of lust? Perhaps lust in a higher ratio is what suppresses the affectionate love?"

I posed this question to Dr. Money, and he replied, "It would be better to do research study and prove it." In fact, I was already on the path of that research. I thought to myself that perhaps I could leave prison and fall in love, but without my paraphilic lust eventually destroying my romantic or marital partnership. I felt optimistic for the first time in many years.

Yes, I could conceal my masochism. But I don't want to go on that way. It hasn't been actuality that has disturbed me, rather it has been my mental reality that has tormented me. I'm caught between two worlds or realms: the socially ideal realm, and my imprinted realm. I cannot choose, for it has been chosen for me, prepubertally. However, even if I weren't criminally responsible, I'm still accountable for my past and present actions.

I pondered, "Someone might read this and mock me unmercifully. You don't want your stoical father or myopic family members to know that you got spanked by a young blonde. Suppose the inmates who know you read this story? You'll never hear the end of their derision. You're already miscast as unmanly by the exaggerative men; this would justify their miscasting."

I had a coping tactic for myself in view of male adulation, with its distortions and exaggerations. I reminded myself I am a man by virtue of my genitalia, and all the rest is stereotype. That seemed a primary defect with all inmates, their distorted stereotypes of maleness.

To continue scientifically, I stood in need of a standard for pairbonded love and pairbonded lust. My criterion for pairbonded love was an affectionate attachment and tender inclination toward a partner. Pairbonded lust would be a longing, eagerness, and inclination for copulation with a partner. In normophilia, these two would coexist. Typically, a person with a paraphilia would have a split of love from lust. In prison an inmate's pairbonded lust holds center stage in his male and female partnerships. It is overactive, primary, coercive, and distorted. Survival with a partner, and in society, however, is dependent upon the modifying influence of a pairbonded love. It is endemic in most inmates to assume that the desire of lust is love. Once I also assumed the same.

I had already accepted the concept that there is a threshold for love pairbonding in the brain's pathways, just as there is a threshold for learning to use a language, in human beings. Now I needed to prove that pairbonded love could develop, or be developed, especially when it seemed inactive, or greatly detached from lust.

At the outset of 1990, the frequency of my paraphilic imagery and its scenarios had diminished. In my case, pairbonded lust is primarily paraphilic lust. I must admit, I missed my ecstatic orgasms with their euphoric afterglow. Meanwhile, I experienced a mental pattern of scenarios that meant much more to me. My imaginal scenarios with spouses were affectionately and tenderly reciprocal. The female actresses of my lovemap knew that I suffered a split of love from lust. In some scenarios, my lovemates had the same split. Increasingly, day after day and scenario after scenario, I watched my self-image participate in pairbonded love. Recurrently, my mind's videotapes rehearsed scenes and scenarios of pairbonded love. But I didn't do anything; rather, my predisposition toward pairbonded love rehearsed me for a future actuality of pairbonded love, which would progressively modify my paraphilic lust. By the end of 1991, my scenarios of imaginal pairbonded love had prevailed over paraphilic lust for two consecutive years.

My manic-depressive or bipolar disorder will always inhabit me. But my mentally rehearsed scenarios of pairbonded love diminished my episodes of despairing depression. Of course, by this period, I had assimilated all the aspects and concepts of Dr. Money's sexosophy. His coping strategies or tactics were achieved with great success. They facilitated living in the most hostile place on earth. Moreover, the paraphilic lust that determined my term in prison no longer dominated my life or pairbonding.

Theoretically, my pairbonded love went into hibernation after the incident with my childhood playmate at three years of age. My lust continued to develop, but without the modifying influence of affectionate love. Loveless lust gained and held center stage for most of my life. By definition, I didn't know that pairbonded love existed, nor that it had a biosocial origin.

Our minds don't always accept or adopt into practice that which we discover or learn. But after I discovered the concept of infant and mother and lover and lover pairbonding, my mind did accept the concept of pairbonded love. Fortunately, there was an appetite for pairbonding that facilitated its acceptance. That concept of pairbonded love has been adopted by my sexual brain, for which it was predisposed, and it now modifies my penile lust and its paraphilic manifestation. My paraphilic lust is now subject to the eroticized convenience of pairbonded love, especially between a reciprocal partner and myself. Presumably, there was a threshold for pairbonded love, which is why it recrudesced.

Yearning to discover more about my impaired love bondedness, I examined my memory and environs. I wondered, "How could I live forty-one years with such a distorted concept of interpersonal or heterosexual love without someone or something correcting me?" I then discovered a major source of misinformation right in front of my eyes: television and the media. With total indifference to the three forms of love, they instruct us to love everything and everyone the same way: as an elevated form of desire, or to like so-and-so very, very much.

All the media messages are contrary to the poetry of love. Television, romantic magazines and novels, erotica, talk shows, the news, misguided parents, religion, misinformed therapists—all are the same. Love, as in the state of being in love, is not merely an active desire, nor is it an altered form of like. It has a biosocial origin conducing partners to an affectionate attachment and tender inclination toward one another as mates, lovers, or spouses. The longings, eagerness, and inclinations of lust are not and should not be misconstrued as pairbonded love. Ideally, two-partnered love and genital lust are coequal and coexistent within an erotic partnership, which might be marital or nonmarital, and also might fit the criterion of pairbondedness as heterosexual, bisexual, or homosexual.

Figuratively speaking, if television and its massive influence had its way, I'd be falling in love with, and reproducing, cereal, sausage, pancakes, pickles, hot dogs, popcorn, bread, cold medicine, houses, cars, boats, trips, toys, eye shadow, makeup, broadcasts, money, murder movies, tools, guns, cups, mugs, coffee, tea, news, tobacco, prescription and nonprescription drugs, games, sports, toothpaste, mouthwash, candy bars, books, magazines, and videotapes. I'd be pansexual if I fell in love with all those products. Properly, I can fall in love only with a person, not a product.

Throughout the six years of examining and researching my own lovemap, I discovered three types of partners with whom I might fall in love. I also discovered how I or anyone falls in love. This was important because I didn't want to become attached to another dominatrix and like a fool to assume it to be love.

It used to be that I'd have to say: I can fall in love with specific adolescent females only. They already exist, in some form, in my sexual brain or lovemap. They await an actual parallel to match their imagery, that is, an actual or objective female who looks similar or exactly like the subjective or composite female residing within my brain's lovemap.

As a result, I used to say: I cannot experience heterosexual love or paraphilic lust for an animate female who is not a reasonable facsimile of an imagined female. I can fall in love with two women at the same time, but never in the same manner. One woman would earn my affectionate or pairbonded love, whereas the other woman would share my pairbonded lust.

There must be an interchange of images to experience the phenomenon of falling in love. I can test and validate my own experience of being in love. The state of love has variables. I have discovered how to predict or estimate the longevity or duration of my own state of love. The imagery and ideation of my mind will shape the love affairs or lust affairs of my life. Love's state can occur not only between the viewer and the view, but also within the viewer only.

I've discovered also that scenarios have been and are staged within my mind anticipating the appropriate actresses. In other words, my mental stage is set, waiting for the typecast character to match my mental casting of that character. When the two merge, an actualized love or lust affair commences, as predisposed, or staged.

I have concluded, from retrospection and introspection, that pairbonded love outlasts pairbonded lust. That's because pairbonded lust is dependent upon genital arousal, but pairbonded love is not. My observation is that pairbonded love provides the attachment for my partner, whereas pairbonded lust facilitates genital ecstasy. A good example of this is Denise, the partner who eventually introduced me to Connie. I was spurred to lust upon my first sighting of her physique. I experienced an affectionate attraction with an overwhelming penile arousal. Then Denise moved. A year later she returned, having gained extra weight and gotten pregnant.

A few months after Denise's baby was born, I took her out to dinner. She longed to behave sexually with me. I had a hard-on from my memory imagery of her. But when I observed the result of her stretched skin and the scar from surgery, my penis deflated. Her form ceased to interchange reciprocally with the imprinting and composite imagery of my lovemap. My pairbonded love for Denise endured, but my pairbonded lust failed.

When I met Connie, my mental stage had already been set for a dominatrix. Figuratively speaking, when I met Connie she said, "I'm the parallel to that dominatrix who looks like me in your mind." Connie didn't possess all of the required characteristics for my ideal dominatrix. But those characteristics she lacked, my vandalized lovemap typecast her as possessing anyway. That miscasting is why our paraphilic partnership eventually failed. Nonetheless, today I have a fondness for her, but no lust whatsoever. She no longer fits the dictates of my vandalized lovemap. Mostly, she's too old. According to the dictates of my ephebophilic lovemap, I can't experience penile arousal for a female who is over thirty. I'm an ephebophile. Incidentally, that is why an older man may leave a marital partnership of ten years. It's not because he is looking for a final fling of romance. It's not because older men invariably seek younger women. It's because of the paraphilia known as ephebophilia. And an ephebophilic lovemap makes one's genital arousal contingent on the youth of the partner.

For six consecutive years, I watched my mental theater. As far as I am concerned, I've discovered the ultimate therapy, especially for the paraphile. It bypasses the phrase: "What's good for you might not be good for me." I believe that my own ideating has produced something as profound for me as was the discovery of the atom for science. The Division of Corrections will lose this occupant forever. Paradoxically, I've discovered the answers to life in prison, a place that resists and discourages self-improvement.

While using my skills as a writer and salesman, I intend to teach my sexosophy to the women of America, and to America's paraphilic males. Why the women? Because women don't have as many paraphilias as men. Furthermore, my sexosophy is based on language, and women don't vulgarize language the way men do. My sexosophy starts with mother and infant. It commences the moment she speaks to her newborn infant. At any age, language and pairbonding are the answers to a better life on earth.

My own discovery, concerning language and pairbonding, now

shares power with my genes and internal chemistries in governing my entire organism, its function and practices. Indeed, my discoveries are now a biological part of me. They cannot be eradicated except by a neurosurgeon's knife.

I work on the assumption that all of the lovemates or lustmates I'll ever meet are already represented in my brain's lovemap, irrespective of whether my lovemap's imagery is paraphilic or nonparaphilic. They are waiting for me to encounter their match, or partial parallel. I discovered this concept during my six years of introspective self-examination.

No potential dominatrix can overwhelm me ever again. I already know what a dominatrix will look like. I am forewarned and protected by an insight along with a precise language to define that insight. My misrelated lust fails to be my primary source of stimulation anymore. Pairbonded love takes its place as my primary source of stimulation— it is waiting to be tested in the man-and-woman world beyond the all-male confinement of an institution that absurdly calls itself correctional.

Formerly, I'd say, "I feel or sense it, but I can't explain it." Subsequently I absorbed the appropriate words from which were made ideas. Those words facilitated my brain's assimilation and comprehension. Now I can avoid the struggling lover's dilemma: How do I really know if what I feel is the state of love? As a result, I'll never be caught in a masquerade of love. If I'm experiencing a partial effect of love's state, I'll know it, for I have the language to define it, and to do so quite precisely.

The language of pairbonded love is curative for the paraphile. Cure cannot be induced solely by medication, however. It must be absorbed by way of the mind into the paraphile's organism.

Glossary

androgyny (*adj.* androgynous): the condition of showing some characteristics of both sexes in body, mind, or behavior.

biastophilia (*adj.* biastophilic): a paraphilia of the sacrificial/expiatory type in which sexuoerotic arousal and facilitation or attainment of orgasm are responsive to and contingent on the surprise attack and continued violent assault of a nonconsenting, terrified, and struggling stranger (from Greek *biastes,* rape or forced violation + *-philia*). Acquiescence on the part of the partner induces a fresh round of threat and violence from the biastophile. Biastophilia may be homosexual as well as heterosexual, but is predominantly the latter, whether the biastophile is male or female. There is no term for the reciprocal paraphilic condition, namely, stage-managing one's own brutal rape by a stranger, which probably exists chiefly in attenuated form and rarely gets transmuted from fantasy into actuality. *Syn.* raptophilia.

chrematistophilia (*adj.* chrematistophilic): a paraphilia of the mercantile/venal type in which sexuoerotic arousal and facilitation or attainment of orgasm are responsive to and contingent on being charged or forced to pay, or being robbed by the sexual partner for sexual services (from Greek *chremistes,* money dealer + *-philia*). There is no technical term for the reciprocal paraphilia condition of enforcing a charge or robbing.

157

coitus or **coition** (*adj.* coital, *adv.* coitally): the sexual act, specifically the taking of the penis into the vagina, or the penetrating of the vagina with the penis; more generally the complete interaction between two sexual partners.

coprophilia (*adj.* coprophilic): a paraphilia of the fetishistic/talismanic type in which sexuoerotic arousal and facilitation or attainment of orgasm are responsive to and contingent on being smeared with and/or ingesting feces (from Greek *kopros*, dung + *-philia*). There is no technical term for the reciprocal paraphilic condition of defecating in the mouth or over the body of the partner.

copulate (*n.* copulation): to couple, join, or unite as in sexual interaction and genital union.

cunnus: the Latin term for the female external genitals; in English, cunt (*adj.* cuntal).

ephebophilia (*adj.* ephebophilic): a paraphilia of the stigmatic/eligibilic type involving attraction to a partner whose age is postpubertally adolescent (from Greek *ephebos*, a postpubertal young person + *-philia*).

erotomania: morbid exaggeration of or preoccupation with sexuoerotic imagery and activity (from Greek *eros*, love + *-mania*, madness).

erotophonophilia: a paraphilia of the sacrificial/expiatory type in which sexuoerotic arousal and facilitation or attainment of orgasm are responsive to and contingent on stage-managing and carrying out the murder of an unsuspecting sexual partner (from Greek *eros*, love + Greek *phonein*, to murder + *-philia*). The erotophonophile's orgasm coincides with the expiration of the partner.

fellatio (*v.* to fellate): erotic stimulation by sucking (from Latin, *fellare*) of the penis with the lips, mouth, tongue, and throat, by a partner of either sex, as a part of normal loveplay, and possibly inducing orgasm.

fugue: an altered state of consciousness in which what is happening now is unrelated to or dissociated from, what had happened before, in the preceding phase of existence; as, for example, in the alternating manifestations of dual or multiple personality (from Latin *fuga*, a flight).

genitalia (*adj.* genital, *adv.* genitally): the sex organs, internal and external. The word is often used to refer to the external organs only. *Syn.* genitals.

gynephilia (*adj.* gynephilic): love of a woman by a man (male gynephilia) or by a woman (female gynephilia). It includes erotosexual bonding.

homicidophilia: *see* erotophonophilia.

hybristophilia (*adj.* hybristophilic): a paraphilia of the marauding/predatory type in which sexuoerotic arousal and facilitation and attainment of orgasm are responsive to and contingent on being with a partner known to have committed an outrage or crime, such as rape, murder, or armed robbery (from Greek *hybridzein,* to commit an outrage against someone + -*philia*). The partner may have served a prison sentence as a convicted criminal, or may be instigated by the hybristophile to commit a crime and so be convicted and sent to prison.

ideation (*adj.* ideational): in mental life, the collective representation of thoughts and ideas presently recognized, recalled from memory, or projected into the future, singly or in combination.

imagery: in mental life, the collective representation of mental images or depictions of anything either perceived (perceptual imagery) or, if not actually present as a sensory stimulus, recognized in memory (memory imagery), or in dream, confabulation, or fantasy (fictive imagery).

imaginal: pertaining to imagination, images, or imagery.

imprinting: developmental learning of a type first brought to scientific attention in studies of animal behavior by ethologists. Imprinting takes place in a given species when behavior phyletically programed into the nervous system of that species requires a matching socioenvironmental stimulus to release it, when the matching must take place during a critical or sensitive developmental period (not before or after), and when, having occurred, the resultant behavior pattern is unusually resistant to extinction. In human beings, native language learning is a manifestation of imprinting.

intersex (*adj.* intersexual): diagnostically a synonym for hermaphroditism, a birth defect in which the genitalia are anatomically ambiguous. As a synonym for heterosexual it means interaction between male and female, as contrasted with intrasexual, within the self.

Jekyll and Hyde: a character with dual personality, the law-abiding Dr. Jekyll and the monstrous Mr. Hyde, created by the author Robert Louis Stevenson.

limerence (*adj.* limerent): a recently coined name (Tennov, 1979) for the experience of having fallen in love and being irrationally and fixatedly love-smitten, irrespective of the degree to which one's love is requited or unrequited.

lovemap: a developmental representation or template in the mind and in the brain depicting the idealized lover, the idealized love affair, and the idealized, program of sexuoerotic activity projected in imagery or actually engaged in with the idealized or actual lover.

loveplay: affectionate play engaged in by lovers and not necessarily including genital juxtaposition.

lovesickness: the personal experience and manifest expression of agony when the partner with whom one has fallen in love is a total mismatch whose response is indifference, or a partial mismatch whose reciprocity is incomplete, deficient, anomalous, or otherwise unsatisfactory.

lust: longing, eagerness, inclination, or sensuous desire; normal sexual desire, or sexual desire stigmatized as degrading passion.

manic-depressive cyclicity: in manic-depressive illness, the repeated sequence of a period of being high (manic) followed by one of being low (depressive).

masochism: a paraphilia of the sacrificial/expiatory type in which sexuoerotic arousal and facilitation or attainment of orgasm are responsive to and contingent on being the recipient of abuse, torture, punishment, discipline, humiliation, obedience, and servitude, variously mixed (named after Leopold von Sacher-Masoch, 1836–1895, Austrian author and masochist). The reciprocal paraphilic condition is sadism.

masturbation fantasy: cognitional rehearsal of erotically stimulating activity that accompanies, and may precede, an episode of masturbation. To the extent that the content of its imagery and ideation, like that of a sleeping dream, has a high degree of autonomy and individual specificity in its power to stimulate genital arousal, it is not voluntarily chosen or preferred.

normophilia (*adj.* normophilic): a condition of being erotosexually in conformity with the standard as dictated by customary, religious, or legal authority (from Latin *normo-* + *-philia*).

pairbonding (*adj.* pairbondant): a condition signifying the reciprocal and mutually interdependent attachment of two individuals, each to the other, for example, the condition that exists between a parent and child (*noun* pairbondship, -ance, -age, the existence of such a condition).

pansexual (*adj.*): expressing sexuality and eroticism in manifold and different ways.

paraphilia (*adj.* paraphilic): a condition occurring in men and women of being compulsively responsive to and obligatively dependent on an unusual and personally or socially unacceptable stimulus, perceived or in the ideation and imagery of fantasy, for optimal initiation and maintenance of erotosexual arousal and the facilitation or attainnent of orgasm (from Greek *para-*, altered + *-philia*). Paraphilic imagery may be replayed in fantasy during solo masturbation or intercourse with a partner. In legal terminology, a paraphilia is a perversion or deviancy; in the vernacular it is kinky or bizarre sex.

paraphiliac: a person with a paraphilia. *Syn.* paraphile.

pedophilia (*adj.* pedophilic): a paraphilia of the stigmatic/eligibilic type in which sexuoerotic arousal and the facilitation or attainment of orgasm in a postpubertal adolescent or adult male or female are responsive to and contingent on having a juvenile partner of prepubertal or peripubertal developmental status (from Greek *paidos,* child + *-philia*). Pedophile relationships may be heterosexual or homosexual or, more rarely, bisexual. They may take place in imagery or actuality, or both.

penis (*adj.* penile): the male urinary and copulatory organ, comprising a root, shaft, and at the extremity, glans penis and foreskin (from Latin, *penis*). The skin-covered shaft or body of the penis consists of two parallel cylindrical bodies, the *corpora cavernosa,* and beneath them, surrounding the urethra, the *corpus spongiosum.* The penis in the male is the homologue of the clitoris in the female.

-philia (adj. -philic): a combining form from Greek *philos,* loving, fond of, having a tendency toward.

pudendum (*pl.* pudenda, *adj.* pudendal): in human beings, especially females, the external genitals.

quim: in its standard usage as a verb, it means to take the penis into the vagina and perform grasping, sliding, and rotating movements on it of varying rhythm, speed, and intensity. As a noun, a quim would be the name of the aforesaid practice.

sadism (*adj.* sadistic): a paraphilia of the sacrificial/expiatory type in which sexuoerotic arousal and facilitation or attainment of orgasm are responsive to and contingent on being the authority who variously imposes abuse, torture, punishment, discipline, humiliation, obedience, and servitude (named after the Marquis de Sade, 1740–1814, French author and sadist). The reciprocal paraphilic condition is masochism.

sexology (*adj.* sexological): the body of knowledge that comprises the science of sex, or, more precisely, the science of the differentiation and dimorphism of sex and of the erotosexual pairbonding of partners. Its primary data are behavioral/psychological and somatic, and its primary organs are the genitalia, the skin, and the brain. The scientific subdivisions of sexology are genetic, morphologic, hormonal, neuroanatomical, neurochemical, pharmacological, behavioral, sociocultural, conceptive-contraceptive, gestational-parturitional, and parental sexology. The life-span subdivisions of sexology are embryonal-fetal, infantile, child, pubertal, adolescent, adult, and gerontal sexology.

sexosophy (*adj.* sexosophical): the body of knowledge that comprises the philosophy, principles, and knowledge that people have about their own personally experienced eroticism and sexuality and that of other people, singly and collectively. It includes values, personal and shared, and it encompasses culturally transmitted value systems. Its subdivisions are historical, regional, ethnic, religious, and developmental or lifespan.

sexual rehearsal play: motions and positions observable in infantile and juvenile play, such as pelvic thrusting and presenting, and coital positioning, that are components of, and prerequisite to, healthy sexuoerotic maturity in human and other primates.

somnophilia (*adj.* somnophilic): the sleeping princess syndrome, a paraphilia of the marauding/predatory type in which erotic arousal and facilitation or attainment of orgasm are responsive to and contingent on intruding on and awakening a sleeping stranger with erotic caresses, including oral sex, not involving force or violence (from Latin *somnus,* sleep + -*philia*).

stigmatophilia (*adj.* stigmatophilic): a paraphilia of the stigmatic/eligibilic type in which sexuoerotic arousal and facilitation or attainment of orgasm are responsive to and contingent on specific features of a partner, for example, one who has been tattooed, scarified, or pierced for the wearing of gold jewelry (bars or rings), especially in the genital region (from Greek *stigma,* mark + -*philia*). The same term applies to the reciprocal paraphilic condition in which the self is similarly decorated.

swive: in its standard usage as a verb it means to put the penis into the vagina and perform sliding movements of varying depth, direction, rhythm, speed, and intensity. As a noun, a swive is the name of the aforesaid practice.

symphorophilia (*adj.* symphorophilic): a paraphilia of the sacrificial/expiatory type in which sexuoerotic arousal and facilitation or attainment of orgasm are responsive to and contingent on stage-managing the possibility of a disaster, such as a conflagration or traffic accident, and watching for it to happen (from Greek *symphora,* disaster + -*philia*). The same term is applied to the reciprocal paraphilic condition in which the person arranges to be at risk as a potential victim of arranged disaster.

threshold: the point, stage, or degree of intensity at which an effect begins to be produced. The lower the threshold, the sooner and more easily does the effect begin.

toucheurism: a paraphilia of the solicitational/allurative type in which sexuoerotic arousal and the facilitation or attainment of orgasm are responsive to and contingent on surreptitiously touching a stranger on an erotic part of the body, particularly the breast, buttocks, or genital area. (from French *toucher,* to touch).

troopbonding (*adj.* troopbondant): a condition signifying the reciprocal allegiances among individuals within an aggregation or cluster in mutual interdependency and, conversely, lack of allegiance toward members of rival aggregates or clusters (*noun* troopbondship, -ance, -age, the existence of such a condition).

vulva (*adj.* vulval, vulvar): the external female genitalia.